NewHope

FOR PEOPLE WITH

Alzheimer's

and Their Caregivers

Other Books in the NEW HOPE Series

New Hope

FOR PEOPLE WITH

Alzheimer's
and Their Caregivers

Porter Shimer

Foreword by Juergen H. A. Bludau, M.D., C.M.D.

Reviewed by Juergen H. A. Bludau, M.D., C.M.D.,
and Avrene L. Brandt, Ph.D.

 THREE RIVERS PRESS
NEW YORK

Published by Three Rivers Press, New York, New York.
Member of the Crown Publishing Group, a division of Random House, Inc.
www.crownpublishing.com

THREE RIVERS PRESS and the Tugboat design are registered trademarks of Random House, Inc.

Originally published by Prima Publishing, Roseville, California, in 2002.

In order to protect their privacy, the names of some individuals cited in this book have been changed.

Interior design by Peri Poloni, Knockout Design
Illustrations by Laurie Baker-McNeile

Printed in the United States of America

Library of Congress Cataloging-in-Publication Data
Shimer, Porter.
   New hope for people with Alzheimer's and their caregivers : your friendly, authoritative guide to the latest in traditional and complementary treatments / Porter Shimer.
      p.   cm.—(New hope)
   Includes bibliographical references and index.
   1. Alzheimer's disease—Treatment—Popular works. 2. Alzheimer's disease—Patients—Care—Popular works. I. Title. II. Series.
RC523.2 .S538   2002
616.8'3106—dc21   2002066343

ISBN 0-7615-3507-1

10 9 8 7 6 5 4 3

First Edition

This book is dedicated not just to the millions of people with Alzheimer's disease, but also to the millions more responsible for their care.

Contents

Foreword

DAY IN AND day out, Alzheimer's disease touches every aspect of the life of both the person with the illness and the caregiver, many times impacting the caregiver's physical and mental health radically. The reality is, the caregiver—whether he or she is a spouse, adult child, relative, or friend—is the single most challenged, misunderstood, and ignored participant in the care and treatment of a person with Alzheimer's disease. In this book, Porter Shimer gives caregivers a guide for their journey along the bumpy, winding, and ever-changing road of dealing with a person who has Alzheimer's. From choosing the right physician to investigating traditional and alternative therapies, Shimer focuses on supplying caregivers with the essential information and tools necessary to navigate the appropriate course for themselves and the loved ones in their care.

The caregiver is the all-important link between the patient and physician. In fact, it is the caregiver who ultimately provides the physician with the most valuable insights and information necessary to reach a diagnosis. It is also the caregiver who makes it possible for his or her loved one to stay in a comfortable home environment for as long as possible, as well as providing support to the medical and nursing staff of a long-term care facility. Unfortunately, the caregiver is often left out of the most crucial decisions and meetings, resulting in a sense of inadequacy, frustration, and overall loss of control. While we search for treatment options and, eventually, the ultimate cure for this devastating disease, we must first and foremost never forget the caregiver.

All the medications, tests, and advances in treatment are of no use if we don't accurately diagnose the disease in the first place, and in many cases this is only made possible by carefully listening to the caregiver; something many physicians fail to do.

I often equate this to a pediatrician diagnosing a 3-year-old without any input from the parent or caregiver. Obviously, this is not the treatment method chosen by pediatricians. Why, then, do physicians treating Alzheimer's disease continue to ignore their most valuable resource for proper diagnosis and treatment? We must look at geriatrics as a mirror image of pediatrics.

Following the diagnosis, identifying the treatment, care, and emotional needs of both the patient and his or her caregiver is crucial. Even more important, the entire health care team must include the caregiver as an essential partner. This allows the caregiver to feel comfortable making decisions for the loved one as the disease progresses and their lives change and evolve.

It is my belief that until we have a cure for Alzheimer's, we must have caregivers! This book provides the information, the insight, the compassion, the hope, and the guidance that all those with the important but difficult job of caring for someone with this disease need.

—Juergen H. A. Bludau, M.D., C.M.D.,
    medical director, Joseph L. Morse Geriatric Center
    and the Institute for Geriatric Research & Training

Acknowledgments

M Y SINCERE THANKS to the following people for making this book possible: Juergen Bludau, Avrene Brandt, Colleen Brooks, Vicky Cahan, Jamie Clark, Wanda Cochran, Martin Diorio, Morris Friedell, Laura Gitlin, Diane Grandstrom, Gail Hamilton, Glenn Hammel, Ann Jones, Daniel Kaufer, Claire Kowalchik, Daniel Kuhn, William Li, Penny Martin, Daryl Miller, Dawn Nelson, Ronald Podell, Paul Raia, Michelle Ritholz, Roger Rosenberg, Jennifer Rovenski, Rick Shaw, Elizabeth Shimer, W. R. Shimer, Gary Small, Andrew Smith, Rudolph Tanzi, Myron Weiner, Ernestine Williams, and David Winston.

Introduction

WHEN RONALD REAGAN announced he had Alzheimer's disease in November 1994, 5 years after the completion of his second term in office, the illness went from relative obscurity to worldwide prominence in the brief time it took the former president to deliver his speech. "I now begin the journey into the sunset of my life," Mr. Reagan said, and with those words a journey began for all of us toward a better understanding and appreciation of this difficult disease.

"The Great Communicator" had done it again, this time alerting the world to an illness with potential for becoming one of the most pressing health problems of the twenty-first century.

Unsustainable is the word David Banks of the Food and Drug Administration's Office of Special Health Issues has used to describe the costs Alzheimer's disease could impose on the U.S. health care system in the years ahead if allowed to continue at its present pace. Already the medical costs of Alzheimer's disease (AD) are $100 billion a year, making the illness our third most costly malady behind only heart disease and cancer. These costs should be considered meager, however, compared to what they've been projected to be as increasing numbers of us succeed at extending our life spans, Banks says. Our odds of developing Alzheimer's reach 1 in 10 by the age of 65 and increase steadily until they are almost 1 in 2 at age 85.

At its current rate, Alzheimer's disease will afflict 14 million Americans—triple its current number—by the middle of this century,

Banks says. This number will be a severe strain not only on the U.S. health care system but also on the financial resources of AD patients and their families. Already the average cost of caring for someone with AD is $12,500 a year even when the patient lives at home, a figure that comes to $174,000 over the course of an average patient's lifetime. When full-time professional care is needed outside the home, the average cost is $42,000 a year but can exceed $70,000 in some areas.

But health officials have recognized this impending crisis, and efforts now are under way to conquer this illness as never before. The Alzheimer's Association alone has awarded more than $100 million in research grants since 1980, and this figure says nothing of the millions more being raised by charities, and the millions on top of that being invested privately by pharmaceutical companies hoping to profit from finding effective treatments and ultimately a cure.

PROGRESS IN THE MAKING

"Big deal," you say? None of this is going to pay off in time to be of much help to you? Don't be so sure. Many experts predict major treatment breakthroughs, and maybe even a cure for Alzheimer's disease, within the next 5 to 10 years. As we'll be seeing in the pages ahead, progress in all areas of Alzheimer's research isn't just moving forward—it's "accelerating," according to the National Institutes of Health in their latest progress report on Alzheimer's disease. "We've been able to learn more about this disease in the past 30 years than has been known in the last 3,000 combined, and much of this in the last few years alone," says Daniel Kaufer, M.D., director of the treatment clinic at the Alzheimer's Research Center at the University of Pittsburgh. "We had our first real breakthrough discovery in 1998, and our knowledge has been advancing exponentially since then."

As a result of these discoveries, we now have medications that can minimize AD's symptoms and possibly even slow its progression, but soon these could be joined by other drugs that will halt or even reverse development of the disease, Dr. Kaufer says.

Also exciting has been evidence that certain "do-it-yourself" approaches also may be effective at combating Alzheimer's disease— things such as diet, exercise, stress control, certain herbal remedies, and even the good old maxim to "use it or lose it." As we'll be seeing in chapter 7, research suggests that keeping our brains active may help strengthen resistance to AD or at least lessen its impact.

We'll be looking at all of these encouraging developments and more in much greater detail as this book unfolds, but as bright as the future may look in terms of treatment and even a cure for Alzheimer's, we still need to learn to deal with the disease in the present. The upcoming miracles of modern medicine aren't going to help get your ailing mother to bed tonight, or you, either, so consider it the primary goal of this book to help us all deal with AD in the here and now.

"With all we've learned about Alzheimer's, there's still no substitute for good old-fashioned TLC when it comes to assuring a patient the best possible quality of life," says Avrene Brandt, Ph.D., a consultant to the Alzheimer's Association and the author of *Caregiver's Reprieve*. What Dr. Brandt is talking about is caregiving—learning to manage this difficult disease on a day-to-day, breakfast-to-bedtime basis.

What will loving caregiving require? A lot, but simply preparing yourself ahead of time will go a long way toward meeting this challenge. Yes, there will be times when you'll feel overwhelmed by your caregiving role, and perhaps as confused and frustrated as the person under your care, but this book will help you get through those times. You're also likely to have more concrete concerns, such as the best options for professional care outside the home when that time comes or how to get your loved one's financial affairs in order—we'll help you with those issues, too.

Our goal in these pages is to help you take care not just of your ailing loved one, in other words, but also yourself. And it's important that you do, because the health of your loved one will depend on it. You may expect to encounter that as a recurring theme throughout this book. Just as Alzheimer's can whittle away at the well-being of those who have it, it can chip away at the well-being of the caregivers, and you'll need to protect yourself from this danger to be of optimal help to the person receiving your care. "Caregivers need to realize they're human, and that caregiving doesn't have to require total self-sacrifice and perfection," Dr. Brandt says. "Each caregiver has a limit to how much he or she can do, and it's important for caregivers to know when this limit has been reached."

WHY THE ROAD CAN BE SO ROUGH

What is it about Alzheimer's disease that can make the caregiving role so challenging?

If you've already had some experience at it, you know. If not, maybe the results of a recent survey will give you a rough idea. A survey done by the Alzheimer's Association in 1996 found that the average amount of time primary AD caregivers said they were spending at their responsibility was 100 hours a week; even caregivers working full-time jobs reported spending an average of 40 hours weekly. Three-quarters of these caregivers reported being regularly deprived of sleep by their duties, not surprisingly, and nearly half confessed to occasionally feeling depressed.[1]

Indeed, as exhausting as taking care of someone with AD can be, its emotional aspects may be the most arresting of all. "It can be very frightening to see a loved one who looks the same but doesn't talk or act the same," says Steven T. Dekosky, M.D., the director of the Alzheimer's Research Center at the University of Pittsburgh. "It frightens people because it represents a loss of self."[2]

Caring for someone with AD also can be scary because of the emotions it arouses in such unexpected ways, says Dr. Brandt. "People may be prepared to experience feelings such as sadness, worry, or frustration as caregivers, but not resentment, jealousy, or anger to the point of rage."

Such negative emotions can occur, however, as your caregiving role may cause you to feel your own life slipping away as you pursue what can feel like a thankless and even useless task. For indeed, people with AD may not always appear as appreciative as they may inwardly feel. They also can act in ways that are totally out of sync not just with their usual personalities but also with what's acceptable by society. Patients may exhibit inappropriate sexual behavior, for example, or make ungrounded accusations, or subject those around them to verbal or even physical abuse. There are biological reasons for these behaviors, as AD can begin to destroy sections of the brain that normally keep such actions repressed, Dr. Brandt says, but the results can be nonetheless challenging to manage from an emotional as well as a physical standpoint.

"We tend to think of Alzheimer's as causing patients to become passive and withdrawn, which it can," Dr. Brandt says. "But it also can cause patients to become extremely anxious as they try to come to grips with their mental declines. The result in some cases can be aggressive or even violent behavior as patients seek an outlet for their frustration and fear."

People with Alzheimer's can also exhibit a strong desire for an independence they can no longer handle, causing them to exhibit "minds of their own," even though those minds may have ceased to function competently long ago. "Patients simply may not want to be helped in ways that we as caregivers want to help them," Dr. Brandt says, "and this can add a tremendous strain to the already very difficult caregiving role."

"COLLATERAL DAMAGE"

You as a caregiver, in other words, are in a position in some ways even more risky than your ailing loved one. If this book had been intended just for the benefit of the estimated five million Americans who suffer from Alzheimer's disease directly, it might have been half as long and twice as easy to write. But its scope has had to be much larger than that because Alzheimer's is a disease much larger than that. The number of people who *have* Alzheimer's disease might be considered just the tip of a much larger iceberg, in fact, given the millions more who, as caregivers, are *affected* by the disease.

"Collateral damage" is the term David Hyde Pierce used recently when speaking before the U.S. Congress to describe the far-reaching effects AD can have on family members and even friends, and it was from personal experience the actor spoke.[3] Hyde Pierce, who plays the eccentric psychiatrist Niles Crane on the popular TV sitcom *Frasier,* was hoping to inspire the federal government to up its ante for AD research, so it wasn't laughs he was looking for as he described how the disease had taken the mind, and eventually the life, of his grandfather several years before. Hyde Pierce spoke of how hard the experience had been not just on him personally but also on his entire family and even friends.

At last count, an estimated 19 million Americans said they have a family member with AD, while 37 million said they know someone with the disease, virtually all of whom stand to be affected by their involvement with AD in some way.

FUEL FOR FAMILY FIRES

As caregivers may begin to feel the strain of their commitment, so, too, can family members who may feel neglected by the person whose time is being so dominated by the caregiving role. Making matters worse, the caregiver may in turn feel guilty for this perceived neglect. "Some very difficult and complicated situations can develop within families when someone in the home has Alzheimer's disease," says Andrew Smith, M.S., a counselor in private practice who specializes in gerontological psychology in Allentown, Pennsylvania. Not only may there be accusations of neglect passed around, but the disease can cause a disruption of basic family structure, Smith says. "Children can find themselves in the uncomfortable position of having to parent their parents, for example, or a once-passive spouse may be forced into a leadership role when the decision maker of old is no longer capable."

Then, too, Alzheimer's can rekindle old fires among family members in situations where it's felt that the responsibilities of caregiving should be shared, Smith adds. "If there are any hot spots that exist between family members, there's a good chance the onset of Alzheimer's will cause them to ignite."

We'll be examining the potential for such family conflicts in greater detail later in this book, and we'll be hearing from experts on how best to deal with them. Should the advice fall short of what you might need, however, never feel afraid or ashamed to seek additional help from a qualified counselor. This is especially true given the adverse effects emotionally volatile environments can have on people with Alzheimer's, Smith says. "Even in later stages of the disease when patients may seem quite unaware, they often are much more cognizant than we may realize and hence vulnerable to the stress they perceive around them."

THE GAP THIS BOOK WILL BRIDGE

If it sounds like a full plate you've got ahead of you as a caregiver for someone with AD, it will be. While we'd like to be able to tell you that all the information you'll be needing in the months and years ahead will be coming readily from your loved one's doctor, a recent survey suggests it may not. A survey of 376 caregivers and 500 primary care physicians sponsored by the Alzheimer's Association found that a "major communication gap" exists between these two groups with respect to the amount of information caregivers say they're receiving regarding Alzheimer's care from their loved ones' doctors.[4]

While most of the doctors surveyed said they readily dispensed the kind of caregiving information families needed at the time of their loved one's diagnosis, between half and three-quarters of the caregivers said the doctors had not. And with respect to medications capable of reducing the symptoms of AD, 80 percent of the doctors surveyed said they believed in the usefulness of such medications, yet only 32 percent of the caregivers said they had even heard about these drugs from their doctors at all.

"Major communication gaps exist between primary care providers and the families of Alzheimer's patients," commented the editors of *Harvard Women's Health Watch* on the results of the survey. "As a result, people with AD may not be receiving early treatments that could slow the progression of the disease, and caregivers may not be getting the help *they* need to cope."[5]

"There's no question it's a problem," says Dr. Kaufer. "Doctors aren't taking the time or using the right language to communicate with caregivers, and caregivers often are simply too overwhelmed at the time of diagnosis to be able to take much of the information in. Caregivers should trust that major efforts already are under way to remedy this situation, however, and we should be seeing a significant improvement soon."

Be that as it may, please trust that this book also will be doing its best to bring this communication gap to a close. We'll be leading you through what it takes to cope with this difficult disease from the time of diagnosis to the time Alzheimer's has run its course, with the goal of keeping *you* well so you can keep your loved one well. Yes, there will be bumps in the road ahead, but as rough as the going may get, trust that if you travel it having gathered all the knowledge you can, you'll have done all that's possible to lessen the burdens of this very demanding disease. Until a cure for AD is found—and scientists feel confident one will be found—quality caregiving supplemented by the most effective and appropriate new treatments is going to have to fill the bill as the closest thing to a "cure" for Alzheimer's that we have. Whether or not our efforts succeed in extending the lives of our loved ones, at least they will make their lives better, and what more treasured service can we offer than that?

IF *YOU* ARE THE PATIENT

But what if your interest in this book is not as a caregiver but rather as a patient or possible patient? What signs does the disease show, how early in the disease do they appear, and what's the best course of action to take?

Trust this book will be answering all of these questions, too. Yes, there are symptoms the disease may show in its early stages, and although they can be subtle at first and easily dismissed or denied, they also can be quite terrifying when they finally appear all too clearly written on the wall.

If you begin experiencing symptoms of what you suspect may be Alzheimer's disease, your first step should be to see your doctor for an evaluation—and yes, even if you're "too young" to have this "old person's" disease. One type of Alzheimer's disease, *familial Alzheimer's disease*, or FAD, can occur in people as young as their 30s or 40s. Although it constitutes only about 5 percent of all Alzheimer's cases, it can occur in genetically susceptible families. The important thing is to be tested, for a very simple reason: At least 60 other medical conditions are capable of causing Alzheimer's-like symptoms, many of which are treatable.

Even if Alzheimer's is diagnosed, moreover, currently available medications—and some 50 to 60 more being tested—can reduce symptoms substantially if the disease is caught in time. You stand only to gain by undergoing the diagnostic process, in other words, and to lose if you do not. Besides, if a former president of the United States can "own up" to having this illness, so can you. Your life can only improve when you do.

CHAPTER 1

Alzheimer's Under the Microscope

❧

*When I try to speak, I see what I'm going to say in my mind,
but then the words turn around and go farther and
farther out of sight, and I can't pull them back.*

—BILL, DIAGNOSED WITH ALZHEIMER'S DISEASE AT AGE 54

MARGARET CAN REMEMBER the color of her first boyfriend's eyes, but not that red means stop or green means go. George used to be very shy, but now is apt to shout obscenities when reminded that soup is easier to eat with a spoon than a fork. And Greta makes toast every morning for her husband, even though he's been dead for over 20 years.

So it goes with Alzheimer's disease (AD), the progressive brain disorder named after the German physician Alois Alzheimer who was first to identify it in 1906. Why does this illness affect the human brain in the strange and unpredictable ways it does, and why does it develop in some people but not others? And how, for that matter, can we distinguish the early stages of Alzheimer's disease from the absentmindedness and other mental miscues that can come naturally as we age?

1

We'll be answering these questions and more in this chapter, and it's important that we do, because with a better understanding of this disease can come better care and more compassion for those who have it. People who have this disease are not crazy, although they may sometimes act that way. Nor are they being willfully disruptive, mistrustful, unappreciative, or unkind—although they may act in these ways, too. People with AD have a brain disorder that alters their normal ways of thinking, and hence of acting, and that they can control no more than a cancer patient can control a tumor.

So settle in and be prepared to learn what makes this disease such a challenge to scientists and caregivers alike. We'll start by going back to the beginning to see how the disease was first discovered. Then we'll go inside the brain of someone with AD to see what the disease actually looks like on a microscopic level. Next we'll look at the symptoms this damage can cause and how we can distinguish these symptoms from what's considered normal for the aging process. Finally, we'll explore what still remains something of a mystery—namely, why this complex disease develops in the first place.

ALZHEIMER'S THROUGH THE AGES

While Alzheimer's place in the medical spotlight has been relatively recent, with research not beginning in earnest until the 1980s, most experts agree the disease has been around for thousands of years—"probably ever since human beings first managed to extend life beyond about six decades," says Daniel Kuhn, M.S.W., the director of education at the Mather Institute on Aging and author of *Alzheimer's Early Stages*.[1] The earliest appearance of what historians believe to be a reference to Alzheimer's disease dates back almost 3,000 years, to ancient Egypt, when symptoms of age-related forgetfulness were described in a religious text known as the *Maxims of Ptah the Holy*. A more detailed description of the disease appears again some 1,100 years later in the writings of a Roman physician named Claudius

Galen, and by the year 1383 in medieval England comes a short test that experts believe doctors used to diagnose the disease. Patients, for example, would be asked:

"What town are you living in?"

"How many days are in a week?"

"How many shillings are in 40 pence?"[2]

Not just doctors of yore, moreover, were noticing age-related mental impairment but also writers and philosophers. Shakespeare, for example, refers to old age as being a time of "childishness" and "oblivion," and Plato is known to have commented to his fellow Greeks that "a man under the influence of old age should not be responsible for his crimes."

Symptoms we now attribute to Alzheimer's disease were, for many centuries, thought to be signs of insanity. The long-awaited light finally

> *Symptoms we now attribute to Alzheimer's disease were, for many centuries, thought to be signs of insanity.*

would be shed on AD in 1906, however, when German physician Alois Alzheimer autopsied the brain of a woman who had been suffering from seemingly age-related memory lapses and other mental impairments (dementia) despite being just 50 years old.

ALZHEIMER'S UNVEILED

The woman's husband, who complained not just of her memory problems but also of her unrelenting and totally unjustified accusations that he was being unfaithful, had brought the woman to Dr. Alzheimer. When Dr. Alzheimer began to study the woman, he indeed had reason to believe that she was not relating to the world in a normal manner. While she could identify everyday objects, she often could not remember them just moments later. She also would use odd phrases such as "milk jug" instead of cup, and sometimes she would stop talking for no apparent reason, suggesting she had lost her train of thought.[3]

Might there be an organic cause, Dr. Alzheimer wondered, something physically wrong with this woman's brain to be making her think and act in these unusual ways?

He would be given a chance to find out a few years later when the woman died, allowing him to make the landmark discovery that would begin our journey toward understanding this complex disease. Using a newly developed high-resolution microscope, Dr. Alzheimer viewed a small section of the woman's brain, unveiling for the first time in history the biological makings of this mysterious disease.

"It is evident that we are dealing with a peculiar, little known disease process," wrote Dr. Alzheimer of the abnormalities he observed in the woman's brain.[4] He had suspected for some time that declines in mental function prior to old age might be due to physical causes, and now he had what appeared to be proof. Before Dr. Alzheimer's discovery, age-related *dementia*—now defined as loss of mental function due to an organic cause—was thought to be a natural consequence of growing older, not unlike facial wrinkles or graying hair. Anything resembling dementia occurring prior to old age was thought to be a form of mental illness. Now, however, it appeared that dementia wasn't so simple, that maybe it could occur prior to old age, and for reasons Dr. Alzheimer had just seen with his microscope.

Within a few years scientists had a name for the condition Dr. Alzheimer had discovered—"presenile dementia of the Alzheimer's type"—and finally an illness that had been plaguing humankind anonymously for millennia had been recognized. The candle of knowledge about AD had been lit, and it continues to shed new light even today as scientists continue their search for treatments, better diagnostic techniques, and a cure.

Plaques and Tangles

What actually had Dr. Alzheimer seen under that microscope to convince him he had in fact discovered a "new" disease?

The illustration below may answer that better than words, but we'll do our best to embellish them nonetheless. Between the nerve cells (neurons) of this woman's brain, Dr. Alzheimer observed what he called "peculiar formations," and within the nerve cells themselves he observed what he termed "dense bundles." The composition of these abnormalities would remain a mystery for many years, as would their role in causing AD's symptoms, but scientists beginning in the mid-1980s would start to learn a great deal about these intruders and the damage they do.

The "peculiar formations" Dr. Alzheimer had observed between the nerve cells in the woman's brain, for example, now are known to consist of a type of protein called *amyloid* that has combined with dead and dying brain cells to form what scientists now call amyloid plaques (see figure 1.1). Not only can these plaques interfere with the normal transmission of nerve impulses within the brain, but they can destroy brain cells within their vicinity, thus fueling the ongoing debate among scientists whether these plaques are more of a cause of AD or an effect.[5]

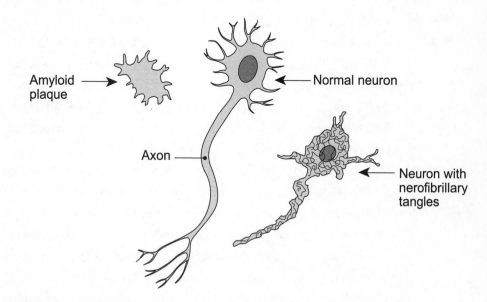

Figure 1.1—*Amyloid Plaques and Neurofibrillary Tangles*

As for the other abnormality Dr. Alzheimer had observed—the "dense bundles" located *within* rather than between the nerve cells of the woman's brain—scientists have found that these also consist partially of dead and dying brain cells plus another type of protein called *tau*. Now known as *neurofibrillary tangles* (see figure 1.1), these growths also eventually destroy brain cells, but in a manner different from AD's amyloid plaques. While the amyloid plaques might be thought of as attacking brain cells from the outside, these tangles do their damage more from the inside. They cause a collapse of the molecular skeleton that neurons rely on not just for structure but also for the transport of nutrients from the body of the cell down to the ends of their tail-like projections called *axons*. This process not only disrupts the ability of neurons to communicate with one another but also eventually causes them to "starve" to death as vital nutrients cease to get distributed throughout the entire cell.[6]

Neurons Bored to Death

But these toxic plaques and tangles aren't the only problems AD poses for brain cells. Some of the brain cells destroyed by these plaques and tangles are responsible for producing important chemicals, called *neurotransmitters*, that brain cells need to communicate with each other. Without adequate levels of these chemicals, brain cells not only have trouble "talking" to one another but also can begin to deteriorate and even die from the biochemical "boredom" that can result. Much like the people they help comprise, brain cells need to stay active to stay healthy, and AD gets in the way.

The result is a very vicious cycle, indeed, whereby a shortage of brain cells leads to a shortage of neurotransmitters, which in turn harms more brain cells, explains Daniel Kaufer, M.D., the director of clinical treatment at the Alzheimer's Research Center at the University of Pittsburgh. Not only does this effect on neurotransmitters help explain why AD doesn't stop once it starts, Dr. Kaufer says, it explains why the cure for AD can't be as simple as replacing the neurotransmitters that AD depletes. "The cure will need to stop the loss of brain cells responsible for this depletion in the first place," he says.

As we'll be seeing in chapter 3, one of the most vital of these neurotransmitters, called *acetylcholine*, has become the focal point of several drugs currently being used to lessen AD's symptoms. The drugs work by inhibiting the action of other chemicals in the brain known to cause acetylcholine to break down, thus helping preserve its presence. Results achieved by these drugs thus far have been encouraging in many patients, Dr. Kaufer says, including improvements in memory and speech as well as the ability to perform certain everyday tasks.

> *Much like the people they help comprise, brain cells need to stay active to stay healthy, and AD gets in the way.*

Whether these drugs help slow progression of the disease or just mask its symptoms is still in question, but in some patients taking the medications, development of symptoms does, in fact, seem to slow down as long as the medications are taken on a daily basis. Norma, for example, whose husband was diagnosed with Alzheimer's 11 years ago at the age of 62, reports that her husband's condition has remained relatively stable for the past several years. "He still has his good days and bad days," Norma says, "but all in all he's been able to remain pretty much the same for the past four or five years, and it's had all of us, his doctors included, very pleasantly surprised."

SYMPTOMS—AS VARIABLE AS THE PEOPLE WHO HAVE THEM

So what are the symptoms Alzheimer's disease is most likely to cause? Maybe you already have an image of someone with the illness in mind—a seemingly lifeless form frozen in a wheelchair, perhaps, or maybe someone wandering down Main Street in bedclothes at midnight.

These scenarios can occur, but they represent extreme cases. It's true that Alzheimer's disease can be quite debilitating in its last stages,

A Day in the Death of a Brain Cell

To get a better understanding of how Alzheimer's disease causes brain cells to die, it helps to understand what brain cells need to live, which they can do for a hundred years or more if all their needs are met. To stay healthy, brain cells need a steady supply of nutrients, they need to be able to repair themselves when they begin to wear down, and they need to stay in communication with one another. The problem with Alzheimer's disease is that it begins to interfere with all three of these needs. Cellular metabolism, cellular repair, and intercellular communication—all begin to break down as the plaques and tangles of AD start to take their toll. What this means for patients, unfortunately, is that once AD starts, it doesn't stop. The insidious nature of this illness is that it has the power to destroy the very mechanisms needed to keep it under control.

Scientists have been making encouraging headway in finding ways to stop this progression, however, which we'll be looking at again in chapter 8 but which we'll mention quickly here to get you thinking in a positive direction. In a groundbreaking series of discoveries made in the 1990s, researchers learned that nerve cells grow tiny projections that sprout from the surface of the cell like blades of grass. In the healthy brain, these growths pose no problem because two types of

and it's also true that as many as 60 percent of patients may experience episodes of wandering from time to time. Just as often, however, the onset of symptoms is gradual and mild, allowing patients to spend their final years in relative peace. "The only thing predictable about this disease is that it's unpredictable," says Avrene Brandt, Ph.D., a consultant to the Alzheimer's Association and the author of *Caregiver's Reprieve*. "Not only can symptoms differ widely between patients, but even the same patient can experience a difference in symptoms from day to day."

enzymes come along, and in a two-step process, clip these growths off in a way that allows them to dissolve harmlessly away.

Not so with Alzheimer's disease, however. For reasons still being studied, a third type of clipping enzyme comes along and makes the all-important first cut at a different spot, not as close to the base of the growth as the first of the other enzymes would. This action in turn changes where the second cut occurs, and therein lies the problem. The clipping created by this second cut does not dissolve harmlessly away but rather lingers to begin combining with other clippings, and the start of an amyloid plaque—and hence Alzheimer's disease—is born.

As we'll be seeing later in this book, scientists currently are working on drugs they hope will prevent this plaque formation by stopping these errant cuts from being made. Some of these medications already have started to be tested in humans. In the words of Kevin Felsenstein, Ph.D., who leads this type of research at Bristol-Meyers, "We're on the verge now of preventing amyloid deposits from building up, inhibiting the production of amyloid, or actually being able to reverse plaque deposition." (See chapters 3 and 8 for more on these exciting developments.)[7]

The reason for this variation remains a mystery but should be considered a testimony to the complexity of the human mind as well as to the complexity of this disease, Dr. Brandt says. What scientists do know about AD, however, is that it typically begins in an area of the brain known as the *hippocampus* (see figure 1.2) responsible for recent memory and learning. From there it moves on to other sections of the brain in charge of such functions as speech, reading, working with numbers, making sound judgments, and coordinating physical movement.

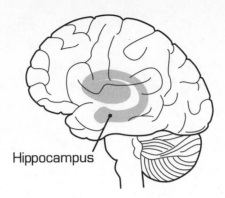

Hippocampus

Figure 1.2—*The Brain*

There is no set pattern to this course of progression, however, and immense variability between people with AD is the result. While some people with AD may be gradually and only mildly affected, for example, others can experience changes that are sudden and quite severe. And while some people may die within just 3 years of being diagnosed, others have been known to live 20 years and even longer. Studies show that the average life expectancy for someone diagnosed with AD is between 8.5 and 10.8 years, depending on the age they're diagnosed, but clearly there's a wide range outside these figures.[8] In the words of Lisa Snyder, L.C.S.W., a social worker for the Alzheimer's Disease Research Center at the University of California at San Diego and author of *Speaking Our Minds*, "a definition of Alzheimer's disease needs to be as varied as the particular course it runs in each person who has it."[9]

This variability should in no way imply that AD does not have very distinct physical causes, however. As we learned earlier and as figure 1.1 shows, the causes of this disease are very real indeed. There can be a tendency sometimes to think of the illness as being "all in the mind," but nothing could be further from the truth. Scientists suspect that the cellular changes in the brain responsible for AD may begin long before symptoms of the disease actually appear—several years, in fact—so the illness certainly has established a firm and very real base before beginning to interfere with a person's life.[10]

Signs to Look For

As much as AD's path can be different for each person, however, scientists have identified certain symptoms as characteristic of the disease that can help loved ones decide whether further testing might be needed. Not all of these symptoms must be present, keep in mind, nor do they need to occur every day for there to be cause for concern. The key is to look for changes from what has been normal in the past. If a loved one is exhibiting any of these symptoms to a degree that is in noticeable contrast to what's been usual for that person, a consultation with your loved one's doctor is a good idea. Currently there's no known cure for AD, but medications are available, as we'll be seeing in chapter 3, that can significantly reduce symptoms if the disease is detected in time.

> *While some people with AD may be gradually and only mildly affected, others can experience changes that are sudden and quite severe.*

Forgetfulness. This is perhaps the most common symptom of AD in its early stages, usually beginning gradually but getting worse over time. A person with AD may misplace things, forget appointments, repeat questions asked just moments earlier, or not be able to recall recent conversations. As the disease progresses, these lapses are apt to become more frequent and severe: the person may forget the names of family members, not be able to identify familiar objects, or begin having trouble with tasks once as familiar as brushing teeth or tying shoes.

Difficulty with language. As recent memory begins to fade, so, too, can the ability to find the appropriate words when speaking, or to hold onto thoughts long enough to form coherent sentences. At first

Alzheimer's at a Glance

The number of people who have AD is just the tip of a much larger iceberg given the millions more the illness affects. This disease burdens family members, friends, coworkers, and even the economy, as the following figures from the Alzheimer's Association attest:

- In addition to the 4 million Americans estimated to have Alzheimer's disease, another 19 million are family members of someone with AD, and nearly twice that many—37 million—say they know someone with the disease.

- Alzheimer's disease afflicts approximately 10 percent of all people over 65 and nearly half of those over 85.

- Women appear to be at a greater risk for developing Alzheimer's disease than men, even when their longer average life span is taken into consideration.

- A rare type of AD called familial Alzheimer's disease (FAD) can develop in people as young as their 30s.

- Complications caused by Alzheimer's disease are estimated to constitute the fourth leading cause of death among adults in the United States behind heart disease, cancer, and stroke.

- People diagnosed with Alzheimer's disease after the age of 65 live an average of 8.5 years while those diagnosed before the age of 65 live an average of 10.8 years. Some people have

this symptom may take the form of midsentence hesitations, but eventually it can lead to sentences having to be aborted altogether, perhaps accompanied by such remarks as, "I forgot what I was going to say." Unlike normal forgetfulness not symptomatic of AD, moreover, whereby the thought eventually returns, the thought lost to Alzheimer's disease usually is lost for good.

been known to live as long as 20 years after being diagnosed, however, while others have died within just 3 years.

- According to some estimates, 60 percent of people with Alzheimer's disease have not yet been diagnosed.

- More than 70 percent of people with AD live at home, and although family and friends provide three-quarters of their care at home, the remainder costs an estimated $12,500 annually.

- Half of all patients in nursing homes have Alzheimer's disease or a related condition.

- The average yearly cost of nursing home care is $42,000 but can exceed $70,000 in some areas.

- The average lifetime cost of caring for someone with AD has been estimated at $174,000.

- Unless a cure or effective preventive strategies are found, the number of people with Alzheimer's disease will more than triple to 14 million within the next 50 years.

- Worldwide, an estimated 22 million people will have AD by the year 2025.

- Alzheimer's disease costs American businesses an estimated $33 billion annually—$26 billion due to lost productivity of caregivers and $7 billion related to costs of long-term care.[11]

Difficulty reading and writing. As language skills wane, the ability to read usually will begin to suffer, too, as the person with AD simply may not be able to retain new information long enough to make sense of what's being conveyed. The ability to write also typically begins to decline as the memory span becomes too short or inconsistent to entertain much less express a logical series of thoughts.

Different Paths for Different People

As proof of just how variable AD can be, consider the following examples of how these two people experienced their first symptoms:

- "At the beginning, I didn't realize what was happening," says Bob, a former mechanical engineer, diagnosed with AD at age 70, who had once helped design lunar modules for NASA. "It was 3 or 4 years before I realized there was a problem. It's not something that comes up and hits you in the head right away."

- Bea would have to disagree. Diagnosed at age 75, Bea had been made aware of her disease in a way that was quite noticeable indeed. While driving into town to get her hair done one day, she failed to make a turn at an intersection and drove straight ahead into oncoming traffic instead. "It was the first time I knew anything was wrong," she would later report. "It was terribly scary," she said, and it would be her last time at the wheel.[12]

Difficulty dealing with numbers. Activities such as adding and subtracting numbers require not just use of memory but also a type of abstract thinking that can begin to suffer in AD's wake. People with AD, as a result, may have difficulty keeping track of their finances, keeping dates straight on the calendar, and eventually even telling time.

Displays of poor judgment. Because making sound judgments requires making sequential connections between a decision and the effects it's likely to have, people with AD frequently will be remiss in this regard as well. They may not see anything incongruous about wearing an overcoat in the summer, for example, or writing checks for money they don't have. This symptom also can lead to rude and inappropriate behavior in public settings as people with AD simply may not have the ability to foresee the consequence of their actions.

Feelings of disorientation. Some research suggests that in addition to disrupting short-term memory, AD may interfere with a person's ability to judge physical distance and space properly, thus leading to feelings of disorientation even in familiar surroundings. Coupled with unpredictable memory lapses, this symptom helps explain why patients can become lost even in settings they've known most of their lives.

> *In addition to disrupting short-term memory, AD may interfere with a person's ability to judge physical distance and space properly, thus leading to feelings of disorientation even in familiar surroundings.*

Failure to recognize familiar people. This can be one of the more upsetting symptoms of AD as people with the illness can forget the names of people, including family members, they've known their entire lives.

Loss of motivation. As people with Alzheimer's disease begin to sense their declining mental skills, they may lose the confidence it takes to remain enthusiastic about things, becoming quiet and withdrawn and forgoing hobbies and perhaps even relationships with friends once important to them. This behavior can lead to serious depression in some cases, which also may need to be treated in conjunction with the AD.

Delusional thinking. Although rare in the early stages of AD, this symptom can become quite prominent as the disease progresses and a person's ability to make logical connections between events and their consequences continues to decline. People with AD may imagine that family members or close friends are stealing from them, or that a spouse is being unfaithful, or that caregivers or medical experts are trying to do them harm.

Changes in sexual habits. Researchers aren't sure yet whether the effect is a physical or psychological reaction to AD, but what they do know is that the disease has been associated with a decrease in sexual interest as well as performance in males and females alike. AD also has been known to boost sexual interest in some cases, however, so clearly more study in this area needs to be done.

Diminished coordination. Because physical coordination depends on a close communication between brain cells and the body's other nerve and muscle cells responsible for movement, physical coordination also can begin to suffer in people with AD, especially as the illness enters its later stages. Complex movements demanding hand–eye coordination such as eating, dressing, handwriting, doing needlework, or driving may be the first to suffer, followed by more general movements required for such activities as climbing stairs or getting out of a chair or bed.

> *As people with Alzheimer's disease begin to sense their declining mental skills, they may lose the confidence it takes to remain enthusiastic about things, becoming quiet and withdrawn.*

A diminished sense of smell. For reasons also needing further study, scientists have found that people with AD exhibit a diminished sense of smell. This shouldn't be considered a definitive sign of AD, as it can be caused by many other factors, but it should serve as an additional piece of evidence nonetheless.

Changes in personality. AD can alter brain function enough to cause profound changes in a person's personality. People once lively and vivacious may begin to lose their spark and become withdrawn, while people who were once shy and reserved may begin to become short-tempered or even hostile. There are biological as well as psychological reasons for these changes, but the changes still can be difficult for family members to understand or accept, especially in the early stages of AD before the disease has been officially diagnosed.

Symptoms Can Be Hard to Accept— and Camouflaged, Too

To know the symptoms of AD, however, is not the same as to acknowledge them, and this point unfortunately goes for family members and people with AD alike, experts warn. The person with Alzheimer's disease may be understandably reluctant to accept the prospect of having a progressive and incurable disease, while the family members may be resistant to face such a grim scenario, as well.

The result can be the proverbial "elephant in the living room" syndrome, says Daniel Kuhn, M.S.W., of the Mather Institute on Aging, whereby major troubles are occurring before anyone is willing to accept the problem for what it is. "Family members may act as if no difficulties exist, or they may minimize their importance. It may even take a crisis before people are awakened to the fact that something isn't right—a fire resulting from food forgotten on the stove, a traffic accident, or utilities being cut off for nonpayment of bills. In some instances it may even take an outsider to recognize that there's a medical problem," Kuhn says.[13]

Making recognition of AD even more difficult is that some people may try to disguise their illness. This behavior might seem surprising in light of the common view that people with AD should lack the cunning for such deceit, but many don't. This isn't to imply that such efforts at cover-up are always conscious, because many times they are not, but deliberate or not, a masking of symptoms can make recognizing AD even more difficult than it already is. "Many people with AD are able to compensate for their impairments, keeping them hidden from family members and even spouses for months or even years," Kuhn says.[14]

> *AD can alter brain function enough to cause profound changes in a person's personality. People once lively and vivacious may begin to lose their spark and become withdrawn, while people who were once shy and reserved may begin to become short-tempered or even hostile.*

People with AD may avoid challenging conversations, for example, or try to steer topics toward the distant past where their recall is apt to be more acute. Or they may relinquish difficult responsibilities such as bill paying or balancing the checkbook to others. If they're still employed, they may go so far as to opt for early retirement rather than have their inadequacies exposed at work. "These are not usually deliberate attempts to deceive but rather instinctive efforts to adapt to changes in memory and thinking," Kuhn says. "It's only human, after all, to want to avoid embarrassment and to be at one's best in everyday situations."[15]

A sense of pride, in other words, often is one of the last human traits that AD erodes.

AD AND DEATH

Although AD is rarely fatal in a direct sense, it always leads to death, if only by indirect means. Since the disease was first identified nearly 100 years ago, in fact, no one is known to have recovered to full health once an accurate diagnosis of AD has been made. In the final stages of the disease, the brain undergoes so much damage that it simply cannot adequately direct all the body's diverse functions, including defense against infections or cancer, or even just the ability to take in adequate amounts of food and water. When the ship in a sense loses its captain, it's only a matter of time before death ensues.

> When people with AD die while still relatively young and active, an accident is often the cause.

The death itself can be from various causes—from germ-driven diseases such as pneumonia, for example, but also malnutrition or dehydration as people with AD may become too feeble, or simply forget to eat or drink during AD's final stages. Heart attacks and strokes also can be common in older people with AD as their growing immobility eventually may compromise the durability of their hearts and lungs.

When people with AD die while still relatively young and active, on the other hand, an accident is often the cause, such as a head injury caused by a fall. Without proper commands from the brain, the body simply becomes vulnerable to a wide variety of mishaps that otherwise might present little danger—climbing stairs, for example, or crossing a street. While Alzheimer's disease might not be what doctors call the

Differences Between Alzheimer's and Aging

While the memory lapses caused by Alzheimer's can be similar to those caused by normal aging, differences do exist. Because no two cases of Alzheimer's disease are exactly alike, however, consider these examples to be generalizations at best:

- While people with age-related memory lapses may forget parts or details of an experience, people with Alzheimer's frequently forget experiences entirely.

- While people with age-related memory problems may forget things temporarily but remember them later, things forgotten by people with Alzheimer's usually are forgotten for good.

- While someone with age-related memory impairment usually is able to follow written and spoken directions, a person with Alzheimer's disease usually is not.

- Self-care rarely is a problem for someone with age-related memory problems, but self-care usually does become progressively more difficult for people with AD.

"immediate" cause of death, therefore, it often qualifies as what they call the "actual" cause of death for having precipitated a fatal event.[16]

THE CAUSES OF AD:
STILL UNCERTAIN AFTER ALL THESE YEARS

As much as scientists have learned about *how* Alzheimer's disease develops, they still have much to learn about *why* it develops. The illness appears to be maddeningly complex, one much like heart disease or cancer that may have as many different combinations of causes as

A Shortage of Glue

Why should it be so characteristic for someone with AD to be able to remember events of the distant past while having trouble recalling events as recent as a sentence they just spoke?

Because Alzheimer's disease attacks first and foremost a part of the brain responsible for taking in and storing new information—the mental processes of which short-term memories are made. "A person with AD, in a sense, loses the 'glue' that enables new information to stick," says Daniel Kuhn.

Spared from memory loss, therefore, are apt to be those recollections of the past that occurred before this important adhesive was lost. "It's the present that poses the greatest challenge for people with AD," says Kuhn. "Compared to that, the past is easy."[17]

people who have the disease. As explained by the National Institute on Aging and the National Institutes of Health in their latest *Progress Report on Alzheimer's Disease*, "Scientists do not yet fully understand what causes AD, but it is clear that it develops as a result of a complex cascade of events that take place in the brain over many years . . . probably as a result of genetic as well as non-genetic factors."[18]

That assessment is based on over 20 years of large-population studies done in the United States as well as Europe and Japan, and while it might give the impression that scientists are discouraged by the immensity of this disease, just the opposite is true. They've never been more intrigued, and this interest has inspired them to search even more intensely for answers. Funding for all aspects of Alzheimer's disease is at an all-time high, and so are scientists' hopes for finding a cure. "We're making progress against this disease as never before," says Daniel Kaufer, M.D., the director of the treatment clinic at the Alzheimer's Research Center at the University of Pittsburgh. "One discovery is leading to another such that our understanding of this disease is growing in an exponential fashion."

Here, thus far, are what scientists feel may be the most influential of AD's possible causes. The first group constitutes risk factors considered to be definite, while those in the second group remain more speculative.

Risk Factors

Scientists aren't ready to call these factors "causes" of AD yet, but they do consider them to be risk factors—circumstances capable of increasing the odds that AD will occur. The more of these risk factors that apply, the greater one's risks for developing AD will be.

> *Funding for all aspects of Alzheimer's disease is at an all-time high, and so are scientists' hopes for finding a cure.*

Advancing Age

Unfair as it may seem, the number one risk factor for developing Alzheimer's disease appears to be life itself. The longer we live, the greater our risk becomes. A rare form of the disease can strike some people as early as their 30s, but the vast majority of people with AD are 65 or older. The Alzheimer's Association reports that our odds of developing Alzheimer's may be as high as one in ten at the age of 65. For those of us lucky enough to make it to our mid-eighties, those odds increase to almost one in two.[19]

A History of AD in the Family

It seems our risks for developing Alzheimer's disease may increase if a first-degree blood relative—meaning a parent or sibling—has developed the disease. Some research suggests having a first-degree relative with AD may increase the risk for developing the disease by as much as twofold, but experts emphasize this in no way guarantees the disease will in fact occur.[20] Our genetic risk, remember, is just part of a constellation of factors contributing to AD that include lifestyle and environmental factors as well. (For an exception to this rule, see side-bar "Sporadic Versus Familial AD" later in this chapter.)

A History of Head Trauma

The human brain is well protected by a skull plus surrounding fluids for a reason: It doesn't like to get knocked around, and professional boxers who wind up with symptoms of dementia are living proof. Not surprisingly, therefore, researchers have found a greater prevalence of AD in people who have suffered some sort of head trauma in their lives, especially if the trauma was severe enough to cause a loss of consciousness.[21] Just how great a risk head trauma poses for AD hasn't been determined, but experts agree that this factor warrants protecting ourselves as well as possible with appropriate headgear when engaging in potentially dangerous leisure-time pursuits.

Lack of Mental Stimulation

The "use it or lose it" adage is one you'll be encountering often in this book, and for good reason: Studies are finding that those of us who "exercise" our brains throughout our lives, either through education or other mental activities, may be more resistant to developing AD as we age than people who do not.[22] Some scientists theorize mental activity may help protect against AD by increasing the number and efficiency of connections between brain cells, thus offering a greater reserve of mental capacity should the disease strike. We'll be exploring this issue in greater detail in later chapters, but take heart for now that there may be more than just enjoyment in playing a musical instrument, writing memoirs, doing crossword puzzles, or reading a good book.

Down's Syndrome

For reasons still being studied, the prevalence of AD is significantly greater among people with Down's syndrome than it is among the general population.[23] Virtually all people who suffer from this form of mental retardation will show some signs of AD upon autopsy at the time of death, suggesting there may be a link between the conditions. For reasons not yet understood, however, many people with Down's syndrome will not exhibit symptoms of Alzheimer's disease during their lifetimes even though autopsies show they have had the disease for many years.

"Possible" Risk Factors

While the increased odds for developing AD associated with the preceding risk factors have been fairly well established, the risks posed by the next set of factors are less certain. Researchers will continue to explore these possible links, however, until their role in the development of AD becomes more clear.

> Researchers have found a greater prevalence of AD in people who have suffered some sort of head trauma in their lives, especially if the trauma was severe enough to cause a loss of consciousness.

Female Gender

Why should more women than men develop AD? That question was given new life in 1999 by a study reporting that the greater prevalence of AD among women held up even when women's greater longevity was accounted for.[24] Some researchers feel declining levels of the female hormone estrogen could play a role, but as we'll be seeing in chapter 8, more work needs to be done before scientists will have a more conclusive answer.

Strokes

Also under investigation is whether people who suffer minor strokes may be at greater risk for developing AD. A recent study of elderly American nuns has suggested that a history of strokes does pose a risk, perhaps by altering normal brain metabolism in some way.[25] The role played by strokes needs to be studied further, but health officials already are advising such stroke-preventive strategies as controlling blood pressure and not smoking as possible ways to avoid AD as well.

Environmental Toxins

For many years exposure to the metal aluminum was suspected of increasing risks of AD, but research reported in 1996 has given scientists reason to consider the evidence weak, at best.[26] Also exonerated in recent years have been the mercury in dental fillings, zinc, and iron.[27] Toxins that *have* been of concern to researchers based on recent findings, however, are certain organic solvents such as benzene and toluene,[28] as well as certain glues, pesticides, and fertilizers for people whose jobs require exposure to these substances on a regular basis.[29] More studies will need to be done, however, before the dangers associated with these compounds can be confirmed.

Smoking

Considering all the other well-documented damage smoking can do to the body, it shouldn't be surprising that AD has been added to the list of risks. The research so far is preliminary but looks strong as evidenced by one study of nearly 7,000 people age 55 and older that found that smokers in the group had increased their risk of developing AD by over 200 percent.[30] Again, however, more research needs to be done, as evidenced by another study reported in 1994 in the *Annals of Epidemiology* that found that smoking might actually help protect against AD. Based on the results of that study, the potential role of nicotine as a memory enhancer currently is being explored.[31]

Free Radicals

Free radicals are mutant molecules that occur as a natural by-product of cellular metabolism, but an accumulation of too many of them in the body over time may lead to tissue damage capable of increasing risks for a wide range of health problems—including AD, many scientists believe.[32] Research currently is under way to explore the potential that certain antioxidant compounds such as vitamins E and C, flavonoids, and carotenoids (found in many fruits and vegetables), estrogen, and the herb *Ginkgo biloba* may have for reducing AD risks.

Diet

If we are what we eat, then our brains may be, too—a logic that has some researchers looking into the role diet may play in the onset of Alzheimer's disease. One study reported in 1994 in the *American Journal of Epidemiology* found that diets high in fat might increase AD risks,[33] while other investigations reported in the *Archives of Neurology* have pointed to shortages of folic acid and vitamin B_{12} as possible contributors to the disease.[34] (For more on the role diet may play in preventing AD, see chapter 7.)

Lack of Exercise

Yes, the warning that "he who rests, rusts" may apply to the brain as well as the brawn. One study reported at the Fiftieth Annual Meeting of the American Academy of Neurology in 1998 found that a group of people with AD had been less active between the ages of 20 and 59 than a group of people free of the disease.[35]

Another study with mice found that physical exercise actually increased the number of neurons in the hippocampus (memory center) of the brain while also enhancing long-term potentiation (LTP), a complex form of electrical activity believed to play an important role in how memories are formed. "Physical activity may be one way to maintain or even improve cognitive function as we age," commented health officials from the National Institute on Aging and National Institutes of Health in their *2000 Progress Report on Alzheimer's Disease* regarding these exciting findings.[36] (For more on AD and exercise, see chapter 7.)

> *Depression is common among people with AD, but is the prevalence more of a cause or an effect?*

Depression

Depression is common among people with AD, but is the prevalence more of a cause or an effect? Scientists currently are exploring this question and already have begun to piece together an answer.

Researchers know, for example, that a shortage of the neurotransmitter serotonin can play a role in both conditions, suggesting depression may be a contributing cause of AD.[37] Doctors also know, however, that depression can be an effect of AD in the sense that many people may become understandably saddened by the prospects of slowly losing their ability to function. Research into this area is continuing, and already many people with AD are being helped by antidepressant medications known as SSRIs that include such brand names as Prozac, Zoloft, Paxil, Luvox, and Celexa.

Sporadic Versus Familial AD

As if scientists didn't have their hands full with just one type of Alzheimer's disease, there appear to be at least three. By far the most common type responsible for an estimated 95 percent of all cases of AD is what doctors call *sporadic Alzheimer's disease* (SAD), so named because it occurs for a variety of undetermined reasons that may in fact be different for each patient.

Far more predictable, because it tends to run in families, is what scientists appropriately have named *familial Alzheimer's disease* (FAD). Not only does this form of AD tend to progress more quickly than the more common type, but in certain rare cases it can occur in what's known as an "early-onset" form and strike people before the age of 60 and sometimes even as early as the age of 30. Far more common, fortunately, is the "late-onset" type of FAD, which doesn't develop until after the age of 60. In both forms of FAD, however, scientists have determined that a defective gene is the culprit, which is why a history of the disease in the family is such a considerable risk. The odds of FAD being inherited from an afflicted parent, some studies suggest, may be as high as 50 percent.

Race and Ethnicity

Might certain racial or ethnic groups be more prone to developing AD than others? Some research suggests yes, although it's not yet known whether genetic or environmental factors have a greater influence. A study reported in 1998 in the *Journal of the American Medical Association*, for example, found a considerably greater prevalence of AD among African Americans and Hispanic Americans of Caribbean origin than among other racial groups—a difference that held up even after disparities in levels of education were accounted for.[38]

Another study, on the other hand, found an uncommonly low rate of AD among a tribe of Cherokee Native Americans living in Oklahoma,[39] and still another found a greater prevalence of AD among Japanese men who had immigrated to Hawaii than in men who had remained in their homeland.[40] Scientists agree that much more research is going to be needed before any helpful knowledge from these findings can be gained.

THE NEXT STEP

So yes, the long-held secrets of this mysterious brain disorder we call Alzheimer's disease are finally being revealed. More work needs to be done, of course, but progress is being made as never before. Let's take a look now at the progress scientists also are making in learning to diagnose this elusive illness, and the importance this holds for maximizing the effectiveness of current as well as future treatments. As with most diseases, the sooner AD is detected, the more successful medical intervention is apt to be.

CHAPTER 2

The Importance
of Diagnosis

I have recently been told that I am one of the millions of Americans who will be afflicted with Alzheimer's disease. . . . I now begin the journey that will lead me into the sunset of my life.

—RONALD REAGAN, IN HIS LETTER TO "MY FELLOW AMERICANS,"
NOVEMBER 5, 1994

THE QUESTION MIGHT seem like a good one: Why put someone through the trouble of being tested for Alzheimer's disease if there's no known cure?

In this chapter we'll see why. We'll see why being tested for AD can be the single most important step against this disease that families can encourage their loved ones to take. There may not be a cure for Alzheimer's disease yet, but treatments are available that can reduce its symptoms and possibly even slow its progress—treatments that need to be started as early as possible to have their best chances of success but that can't begin, of course, until a diagnosis of AD is made. There's also an approximately one-in-five chance that the diagnostic process will show that AD is not even the problem at hand.

Symptoms similar to those of Alzheimer's disease can be caused by over 60 other medical conditions, roughly half of which *can* be cured, so we should see diagnosis as worth the time and effort based on those odds alone.

Perhaps the most compelling reasons for encouraging a loved one to be tested for Alzheimer's disease have to do with emotional issues and something called "the truth." Not until the truth is known can a daughter understand why her once loving father no longer calls. Not until the truth is known can a wife understand why her husband of over 40 years is suddenly accusing her of being unfaithful. Not until the truth is known can a 6-year-old understand why her grandpa forgets not just her birthday now but also her name.

Alzheimer's disease doesn't damage just brain cells, you see. It can damage behavior, and hence people's feelings, and only by way of the truth learned through diagnosis can this damage be controlled. A diagnosis allows for confusion to give way to understanding, for conflict to give way to compassion, and for the nurturing environment that's so important for people with this illness finally to begin.

THE BUCK STOPS HERE

Where does responsibility for initiating this all-important step in the treatment of AD lie? Not with the people who have AD, for reasons that define the disease, and not with medical experts, who simply cannot be present to observe what needs to be observed. The "buck" needs to stop right here, with people like you—the family members, spouses, and close friends who are in a position to observe this illness up close and personally. Not only will you need to observe your loved one, however; you'll need to evaluate what you observe, arrive at a decision based on these observations, and then announce this decision to your loved one in a way that's going to encourage him or her to comply.

It's a tremendous amount of responsibility, which is why we'll be giving you all the help we can in this chapter. From recognizing AD's earliest signs to giving your loved one the right kind of pep talk should a diagnosis appear called for, we'll take you step by step through this critical early stage. If families can't identify the early warning signs of this disease, after all, doctors can't treat it, researchers can't adequately study it, and fund-raisers can't know the magnitude of the challenges AD poses. Scientists' future success against AD, therefore, is going to depend on the success that people like you have right here and right now.

> *You'll need to evaluate what you observe, arrive at a decision based on these observations, and then announce this decision to your loved one in a way that's going to encourage him or her to comply.*

So let's see how this all-important "round one" in the fight against AD can be won. A good place to start is with an understanding of why the illness can be so tough to pin down in the first place.

THE DISEASE WITH A DOUBLE EDGE

If Alzheimer's were a disease that would have the courtesy to introduce itself as formally as most illnesses do, recognizing AD might not be so difficult. But Alzheimer's disease is sneaky, taking years or perhaps even decades to erode the brain's delicate infrastructure before making itself known. Even when the illness does announce itself, its first signs can be so subtle as to be written off as due to stress, fatigue, a bad day, or just another "senior moment." As David Shenk writes in his excellent book on AD, *The Forgetting*, "The disease is so gradual in its progression that it has come to be formally defined by this insidiousness."[1] Doctors now consider this slow-motion onset to be so characteristic of AD, in fact, that it helps them distinguish the illness from other faster-developing dementias, such as those caused by brain tumors, thyroid problems, vitamin deficiencies, or strokes.

As helpful as this slow onset may be for doctors trying to diagnose the illness, however, it can be hellish for loved ones trying to cope with it. "With something like a heart attack or stroke, everybody knows right away what the problem is, and all the right emotions and care can pretty quickly fall into place," says Ronald Podell, M.D., director of the Westbridge Psychiatric Medical Group in Los Angeles.

Not so with Alzheimer's disease. A person's behavior can be a source of confusion and emotional turmoil from the moment symptoms appear, but then it may go on for months or even years before anybody suspects that a physical disease could be the cause. And people

A Word on *Dementia*

You'll be seeing and hearing the word *dementia* often in your dealings with Alzheimer's disease, so a quick explanation is in order. The medical profession uses this word to describe any condition whereby mental impairment has been brought on by *physical* causes. Derived from two Latin words—*de,* which means "away," and *mentia,* which means "mind"—dementia is just that: a condition whereby someone's mental capacities have gone away.

Important to remember, however, is that this "going away" has happened for physical reasons in dementia. This point helps doctors distinguish dementias from murkier conditions more rooted in the psyche, such as schizophrenia and other psychoses that qualify as forms of mental illness. This physical aspect of AD is critical to keep in mind, because while the disease can affect behavior in ways that may appear to reflect psychological instability, the illness is first and foremost a physical one, brought on by the death of brain cells plus a shortage of chemicals (neurotransmitters) needed to keep those cells both active and alive. For this reason, the word *dementia* should not be confused with the word *demented,* which not only implies a psychological illness but has unfavorable moral connotations as well.

can be more than just forgetful, Dr. Podell points out. "Patients sometimes can be mistrustful, accusatory, or even mean, thus giving the disease a kind of double edge that can hurt more than just its victims," he says. "It can hurt those who love those victims, too."

ENDING THE IGNORANCE

But why should Alzheimer's disease cause people to become mistrustful or even aggressive and mean-spirited if it's in fact making them less mentally acute?

"Because it's making them afraid," says Andrew Smith, M.S., a psychotherapist from Allentown, Pennsylvania, who specializes in anxiety disorders in the elderly. "The world of the Alzheimer's patient is one that's forever changing, forever becoming less familiar, and that can be very frightening," Smith says. "Imagine how you'd feel if you sensed you were losing your ability to understand the world as you once knew it, or to think clearly, or to communicate in ways you've been used to your entire life. The onset of Alzheimer's disease can be a very traumatic experience."

With a diagnosis, family members can begin to understand and sympathize with this fear and eventually learn to help make life less threatening for their loved one, Smith says. "Diagnosis can be a kind of ray of light that brings an end to the ignorance and helps guide families in so many ways. It often brings a sense of relief, in fact, as families learn that what they're dealing with is not a mental but rather a physical disease that they can unite against as a team. A diagnosis of Alzheimer's disease actually can be a very unifying force."

It also, however, can be a divisive force for families already at odds over other issues. Decisions about the sharing of caregiving duties and financial responsibilities may cause existing riffs to widen even

> *With a diagnosis, family members can begin to understand and sympathize with this fear and eventually learn to help make life less threatening for their loved one.*

more. Such issues are something family members need to anticipate and minimize as much as possible for the good of the person with AD and the family alike.

We'll be looking more closely at the importance of family unity in dealing with AD, but for now, suffice it to say that while a positive diagnosis of AD can challenge this unity, such a diagnosis also can help strengthen families by establishing a common goal. Strong families generally will grow even stronger in the presence of this disease, Smith says, but weaker families can grow stronger in its presence, too, provided they're willing to address what's made them weak in the first place.

A TIME FOR WATCHFUL WAITING

So diagnosis can offer a lot. By declaring the enemy, a diagnosis of AD can help the person with Alzheimer's and their families wage the right kind of war—not one directed at each other but, rather, one directed at the disease. Just because encouraging a loved one to be diagnosed is the right thing to do, however, doesn't make it easy. Evidence needs to be gathered, a doctor needs to be consulted, and—the hardest part of all—the announcement must be made to the person that testing is deemed necessary. No wonder families tend to drag their feet.

"Families almost always intervene too late," says Frena Gray-Davidson, the director of SHACTI (Self-Help Alzheimer's Caregivers' Training and Information) and author of *The Alzheimer's Sourcebook for Caregivers* and *Alzheimer's Disease: Frequently Asked Questions.* Even when family members do recognize there's a problem, they often hesitate to interfere, she adds. This approach not only paves the way for greater problems in the future but can make for problems in the present. "People with AD simply cannot run their own lives, and it is not an act of kindness to allow them to attempt to do so," Gray-Davidson says.[2]

But just as doing too little too late against AD has its dangers, so does trying to do too much too soon. To attempt to take total control over the life of someone in the early stages of this illness does a disservice to the person with AD and the potential caregiver alike. The former is likely to resist the attempt at control, and the latter is likely to resent this resistance, resulting in ill feelings all around.

What's needed during this difficult time when AD may be evident but not obvious is a period of watchful waiting, Gray-Davidson says. This period can be difficult, because it's natural to want to take action against something we perceive to be a threat, but it's important for family members of people with AD to take time to assess the magnitude of the problem adequately. Gray-Davidson quotes a Buddhist monk when she advises family members how to deal with this difficult time of gathering evidence before informing a loved one a diagnosis is in order: "Don't just do something—sit there."[3]

What's needed during this difficult time when AD may be evident but not obvious is a period of watchful waiting.

Yes, for the time we need to watch more and do less. "This means not trying to force the person to admit, confess, or agree there is something wrong," Gray-Davidson says. "It means being actively kind in order to create a sense of trust that might allow the person finally to share what they're going through."[4] The more we can get our loved ones to open up about the problems they're experiencing, after all, the better we can feel about suggesting that something be done.

DECISION MAKING, FAMILY-STYLE

In addition to being based on as much evidence as possible, the decision to have a loved one tested for AD should be as democratic as possible, including opinions from as many family members and friends as are willing to voice their views. Not only does this strategy share responsibility for the decision, but also it makes for the best chances that the correct decision will be made. "This is a case where several heads really can be better than one," says Dr. Podell.

"Alzheimer's can be so slow and subtle to develop that a variety of opinions can help get the truest picture of what's really going on."

Don't be afraid to include people outside the family in this decision-making process, Dr. Podell says. Outside opinions sometimes can be even more valuable than inside ones because they have an advantage of perspective. "Alzheimer's is an illness with an uncanny ability to dupe those closest to it," Dr. Podell says. "The changes it causes can be so gradual as to be virtually undetectable by those who are around a person with the illness every day."

Don't expect Mom, in other words, to be the best judge of how well Dad is doing. Blinded by more than just familiarity, people emotionally attached to people with AD may want to deny the illness for much the same reasons as the person with Alzheimer's, Dr. Podell says. The denial attempts to protect not only the person with AD, moreover, but also the person doing the denying by attempting to preserve the relationship against changes that a positive diagnosis might bring. "To lose a life-long partner to a nursing home," Dr. Podell says, "can be paramount to losing life itself."

Outsiders Welcome

What such intrafamilial psychosocial complexities amount to is simply this: The ideal decision-making process should include input from not just immediate family members but also friends or even casual acquaintances who may bring an objectivity that emotionally vested family members may not. If your loved one has card-playing friends, a favorite hairdresser or mechanic, or golf or tennis buddies, it certainly couldn't hurt to add their input.

"Objectivity is important, because this can be such a subjective disease," Dr. Podell says. "Sometimes it takes outsiders to see what family members cannot." Behaviors being caused by Alzheimer's may even start to be considered simply part of the person's aging personality, Dr. Podell says. "'Mom's got those 200 cans of soup under her bed because she liked to collect stamps as a kid'—that kind of thing," he explains.

For example, Denise, a 38-year-old mother of three, tells the story of her father, who evidently had been living with Alzheimer's disease for several years before a friend of his finally alerted her father's doctor that something might be wrong. "Dad had always been kind of a loner anyway, so I figured he was just getting older and more set in his ways," Denise says. "He seemed to like living alone and was getting by okay, so I figured I'd just leave well enough alone."

But then "well enough" got bad. "I get this phone call one day from his doctor's office that not only has Dad fallen and broken his hip," Denise says, "he's got Alzheimer's disease. I was devastated. How could I have been so blind?"

SIGNS TO LOOK FOR

What sort of signs might have alerted Denise to her father's condition, and what sort of signs should you and your decision-making team be looking to discuss when you convene to evaluate your own loved one's state?

We've mentioned the major symptoms of AD in chapter 1, but listed in this section are some finer gradations to aid your decision-making process. Generally speaking, what should be cause for concern are behaviors or incidents that represent a decline in a person's ability to think or communicate as effectively as had been normal before symptoms began to appear. This tip might sound so vague as to be useless, but to be much more specific would do an injustice to the disease. This is an illness, remember, with all the complexity of the organ it afflicts. As Lisa Snyder, L.S.W., of the Alzheimer's Research Center at the University of California at San Diego writes in her touching and inspirational book *Speaking Our Minds*, "A personal definition of Alzheimer's disease needs to be as varied as the disease itself—as unique as the particular course it runs in each person who has it."[5]

> *The ideal decision-making process should include input from not just immediate family members but also friends or even casual acquaintances who may bring an objectivity that emotionally vested family members may not.*

Keep that in mind as you peruse this list. Your loved one's illness could be manifesting itself in ways the list does not include. More than any particular behaviors, the important thing is to look for *changes* in behavior—actions or incidents that represent a departure from what has been normal for the person in the past.

> *What should be cause for concern are behaviors or incidents that represent a decline in a person's ability to think or communicate as effectively as had been normal before symptoms began to appear.*

The issues of frequency and degree also should be considered when gauging our concerns, says Steven T. DeKosky, M.D., the director of the Alzheimer's Research Center at the University of Pittsburgh. This point means considering "the functional consequences" of the person's behaviors, he explains. "If Mom forgets where she parked the car at the mall, that's probably not cause for concern. But if she winds up having to walk home from the mall because she forgot she took the car at all, that's a different story."[6]

Here are other potentially meaningful signs to look for:

- Difficulty following through with projects
- A decrease in concern over neatness, hygiene, or appearance
- A suspicious or fearful nature of others for no legitimate reason
- Uncharacteristic emotional outbursts
- Episodes of alcohol or other substance abuse not consistent with previous behavior
- Periods of acting sad or withdrawn for no apparent reason
- A diminished ability to deal with financial matters such as keeping a checking account balanced or paying bills
- A reduction in social activities with friends
- A reduced interest in get-togethers with family members
- A tendency to want to converse about events from the distant rather than recent past

- Exaggerated emotional responses out of proportion to the precipitating events

- A longer sleep time in the mornings, uncharacteristic daytime naps, or a change in sleeping patterns in general

- An increase in household mishaps such as burning meals when cooking or leaving appliances on such as irons and hair dryers

- Illogical thought patterns that fail to make proper connections between cause and effect

- Uncharacteristic auto accidents

AND IF TESTING IS INDICATED?

So what if a few of these symptoms are ringing some fairly loud bells? We wish we could be specific and say that there's a definite number of signs that need to be present for testing to be justified, but, again, the complexity and variability of this illness prevent that. Experts do agree, however, that the existence of more than two or three of these symptoms could indicate a problem. If you're uncertain, consult with your loved one's doctor. Explain the symptoms you've been noticing and for how long, and be ready to answer questions the doctor might have about medications your loved one is taking as well as past illnesses and whether the family has a history of Alzheimer's. If the doctor believes testing for Alzheimer's disease is in order, then the next step is the most important—and maybe the most difficult of all. How, after all, do you tell your dad, say, that he needs to be tested for a disease that is causing him, in essence, to lose his mind?

You don't even come close. "You don't even need to mention Alzheimer's disease at all, in fact, and probably shouldn't unless the patient brings it up," says Rick Shaw, Ph.D., the director of psychology at the Good Shepherd Home in Allentown, Pennsylvania. "The goal at the beginning is simply to get the patient to their primary care physician for a checkup, and nothing more specific than that needs to be expressed."

Could the Nose Know?

Along with memory glitches and lost trains of thought, it seems a diminished sense of smell might also be symptomatic of Alzheimer's disease, and this symptom could even help doctors predict the disease prior to its actual onset. The seemingly unlikely connection, reported in the *American Journal of Psychiatry* in September 2000, was discovered by scientists from the Columbia Presbyterian Medical Center in New York after they gave a "scratch and sniff" test to elderly people who were suffering from mild cognitive impairment, but not Alzheimer's disease. Of the 30 people who did the best on the test, none went on to develop AD when tested 20 months later. Of 47 people who had done poorly on the test, however, 19 went on to develop AD. Even more interestingly, 16 of the 19 people who developed AD said they thought they had done well on the smell test. A diminished ability to smell, therefore, combined with a diminished ability to recognize this inability may be a considerable risk factor Alzheimer's disease, the scientists concluded.[7]

Dr. Podell agrees. "This is not a time to be listing the top 10 stupid things your loved one has done in the past week. You'll be speaking to someone, after all, who already is feeling afraid and confused and doesn't need insult added to injury."

Your goal at this stage should be simply to broach the subject of diagnosis in as nonjudgmental, nonthreatening, and *positive* a way as possible. Tell your loved one that many conditions—over 60, in fact—could be the cause of what he or she is experiencing and that many of these conditions are very "fixable." Explain that even something as simple as a nutritional deficiency or adverse reaction to a medication could be causing the symptoms.

Let Kindness Be Your Guide

Above all, avoid sounding critical or passing judgment in this first meeting, the experts say. Express concern; be kind. Say that you and other family members have been noticing certain things like forgetfulness or moodiness and have been wondering whether maybe your loved one has been noticing them, too. This approach opens the topic up for discussion instead of forcing the person immediately to defend him- or herself.

> *Your goal at this stage should be simply to broach the subject of diagnosis in as nonjudgmental, nonthreatening, and positive a way as possible.*

"Another good approach can be simply to ask questions," says Dr. Brandt. "Ask how the person has been feeling. Ask if he or she has been noticing any changes in things such as the ability to concentrate, or read, or express thoughts. Ask if any activities such as driving, using a computer, or paying bills have been presenting unusual difficulties lately. The idea is to get a discussion going about *possible* problems instead of announcing that it's been decided that a problem already exists." At this point, remember, a diagnosis has not yet been made, and you really *don't* know whether Alzheimer's disease is your loved one's problem. So act this way. If you assume nothing is seriously wrong with your loved one until you learn otherwise, your loved one will have a better chance of feeling this way, too.

Also, you can simply recommend that it's time for a physical checkup, regardless of symptoms, says Ernestine Williams, M.S.W., the director of the Alzheimer's Association multicultural outreach program in Philadelphia. "Many times people showing symptoms of dementia are overdue for a general medical evaluation anyway, so this can be a nonthreatening way to get the diagnostic process started.

From a general physical exam, it usually will become apparent if a possibility of Alzheimer's exists, and required testing can be picked up from there," Williams says.

A Last Resort

What if even the most positive approach you can muster falls on deaf ears? First, don't be surprised, these experts warn. Not only is it a natural human reaction to be in a state of denial about a condition as potentially serious as AD, but denial is especially characteristic of the generation that currently most often has the illness. Many of the people now developing AD are people who've been hardened by the Great Depression and two world wars, Gray-Davidson points out. For these people, silence is safety, while it also connotes strength. They may believe that an illness should be no one's concern but one's own, and the problem ignored is the one more apt to go away.[8]

If you encounter this attitude, your next step should be to ask your loved one's doctor to pick up the ball, especially if the relationship between the two has been a good one. Often the additional element of authority that comes from a doctor can provide the needed weight.

As symptoms progress, your loved one may become more receptive to the ideas of diagnosis and treatment, which you should keep open as topics of discussion.

And if even this fails? Then you may have done all you can, the experts say. By law, no one over the age of 14 may be coerced into medical treatment against his or her will, so unless you're prepared to argue for power of attorney or legal guardianship of your loved one in a court of law, you've gone as far as you can go. Even if these legal prerogatives are granted, you still cannot physically force your loved one to undergo the elaborate testing procedures without his or her cooperation. These are mandates that grant power over legal and financial issues, but they would be of no help in coercing your loved one physically to do something unwillingly.

Reaching this sort of impasse needn't mean abandoning your mission, however. You just may need to put it on hold. As symptoms progress, your loved one may become more receptive to the ideas of diagnosis and treatment, which you should keep open as topics of discussion. As Ben Franklin wisely observed, "Small strokes fell great oaks." Keep chipping away, because AD can be a great oak indeed.

Tips for Getting Diagnosis Under Way

As much sense as diagnosis makes, however, getting a loved one to agree to the process can be easier said than done. You need to convince your loved one first that a problem exists and then that a diagnosis is the best way to handle it. The first of these tasks may be met with denial, and the second may be countered with the flawed logic that ignoring something helps it go away or that doctors usually only do more harm than good.

Given these challenges, we've compiled some general tips, followed by some more specific suggestions should you still feel unsure of how to put these ideas into actual words. Notice with all these suggestions—the general as well as the specific—that optimism rules. It's important to impress on your loved one that whatever is found to be causing the symptoms, seeing a doctor can only make it better rather than worse.

> *It's important to impress on your loved one that whatever is found to be causing the symptoms, seeing a doctor can only make it better rather than worse.*

Push less; care more. Persuading someone to be tested for Alzheimer's disease can be much like trying to handle a bar of wet soap: the harder you try, the more your goal is apt to slip away. Be gentle in your suggestions, explaining that there's a reasonable chance that the problems your loved one is experiencing could be due to something treatable, but only by way of diagnosis can this be found out.

Make it a group decision. Several heads can be better than one, especially when it comes to making difficult medical decisions such as

Evidence of AD Determined by Phone

The system isn't up and running yet, but it could be soon, thanks to the encouraging results of a study by James C. Mundt, M.D., from Healthcare Technology Systems, Inc., in Madison, Wisconsin. Funded by the National Institute on Aging and reported in the November 12 issue of the *Archives of Internal Medicine*, Dr. Mundt's study found that a computerized, voice-driven phone system that asked a series of interactive questions (such as "press the '7' key three times" and "spell the word 'fun' using the number keys") was able to identify people with Alzheimer's disease with an accuracy rate of 82 percent. While this figure is impressive, Dr. Mundt stresses that his system would not be appropriate for diagnosing Alzheimer's disease but rather only for identifying people showing enough evidence of the disease to warrant further examination. Similar phone systems currently are being used to screen people for depression, anxiety, high blood pressure, and substance abuse, Dr. Mundt notes. (Check with your local chapter of the Alzheimer's Association ([800] 272-3900) for information regarding when such a system might be available in your area.)[9]

this one. As suggested earlier, call a meeting of all interested family members and possibly even close friends—or organize a conference call if location is a problem—and discuss what each of you has found to be behaviors or incidents worthy of concern.

Ask for your loved one's input. This approach is often overlooked, but it can be vitally influential in a positive outcome, says Dr. Brandt. Ask your loved one how he or she has been feeling. Has the person been noticing any memory problems, or feelings of confusion, or difficulty in doing any mental tasks that once were routine? "By asking in a caring way, you present the situation in a much less threatening way," Dr. Brandt says. By announcing to your loved one deficiencies *you* have noticed, you risk obfuscating the truth by forcing him or her into a position of self-defense.

Explain there's everything to be gained. While the reasons for diagnosis usually make abundant sense to family members, they often will escape the person needing to be diagnosed, so some friendly persuasion may be required before this all-important first step toward treatment can be made. As clearly as possible, try to explain to your loved one that there simply is nothing to be lost by diagnosis and everything to be gained. Explain that diagnosis not only can detect causes of mental impairment that can be eliminated entirely, such as vitamin deficiencies or adverse medication reactions, but also can improve chances for successful treatment even if AD does exist.

> *A*lthough it's impossible to predict how much success any given person will experience from treatment once a diagnosis has been made, it certainly can't hurt to paint as positive a picture as possible about the improvement your loved one might expect.

Talk of treatment success. Although it's impossible to predict how much success any given person will experience from treatment once a diagnosis has been made, it certainly can't hurt to paint as positive a picture as possible about the improvement your loved one might expect. This doesn't mean making outlandishly false promises, but it does mean sounding optimistic. As we'll be seeing throughout this book, some individuals respond to the newest AD medications remarkably well, especially in the areas of memory and speech. Other medications are available to help with symptoms of AD such as depression, aggressiveness, and wandering.

Make for a path of least resistance. This means setting up the appointment for the diagnosis at a time convenient for the person being evaluated and also being prepared to supply transportation to and from the appointment if necessary. It also can be a good idea to accompany your loved one during the diagnostic tests themselves to help ease fears.

Don't be afraid to ask for help. Ask your loved one's doctor or call the Alzheimer's Association's HELPLINE ([800] 559-0404) about how to get in touch with a social worker who can help you explain to your loved one the need for a diagnosis. The Alzheimer's Association also can give you information on how to become the member of a caregiver's support group where you can gain valuable caregiving advice once your loved one's diagnosis has been made.

If these tips have you feeling you still might be a bit lost for words when it comes time to speak with your loved one about being tested for AD, here are some actual presentations to help you even more. Notice that in addition to stressing the positive aspects of having a diagnosis, each approach employs questions that express concern and invite the person to open up instead of making judgments that force the respondent into a position of self-defense:

- "I'm not saying this to be critical, because I'm sure I do it, too, but have you noticed that when you ask a question, you'll often ask it again just a few minutes later? It's probably nothing serious, but wouldn't you agree that it certainly couldn't hurt to get it checked out just in case? Doctors now have medications that can help with memory problems, and I've heard they work pretty well."

- "I know you can have your 'senior moments,' as you call them, but does it worry you that you've been forgetful more than usual lately? Memory problems can be caused by a lot of things doctors can treat, you know, so would you mind if we made an appointment to see your doctor? You're due for a checkup anyway, you know."

- "I've been worried about how withdrawn you've seemed lately. Is it anything you'd like to talk about or I can help with? It could be due to a medical problem that can be treated, you know, or something really simple like a problem with one of your medications, so would you mind if we made an appointment to get it checked out?"

HOW SCIENCE DECIDES

As futile as diagnosing Alzheimer's disease might seem, we should see it as just the opposite. We should see it as the most important step we can make to assure the optimal well-being of everyone concerned with this illness. "There simply is everything to be gained by the diagnostic process and nothing to be lost," says the Alzheimer's Association's Ernestine Williams. "People with AD benefit by gaining access to the best care, and families benefit by learning what they're up against. It's a win-win for everybody and probably the single most important step against Alzheimer's disease that family members can make.

That said, let's take a look at what this all-important first step toward optimal treatment of AD involves. It can be a fairly elaborate undertaking, requiring several days and visits to more than one location unless a clinic specializing in AD is put in charge. The diagnosis also may take a few weeks to be reached—which is not surprising, however, given that the results of as many as six different types of tests, done by several different types of medical experts, may need to be evaluated.

Why so many tests for just one disease? Because many other medical conditions need to be ruled out before even a "probable" diagnosis can be made. Aside from a new imaging technique still in experimental stages (see chapter 8), only a biopsy of the brain done after death can determine AD for sure, so until better diagnostic techniques are perfected, this battery of tests will have to do. The degree of accuracy achieved by this method in the hands of a qualified diagnostic team, however, is very good—about 90 percent.

> Why so many tests for just one disease? Because many other medical conditions need to be ruled out before even a "probable" diagnosis can be made.

If you're not comfortable with this percentage or are unhappy with the outcome of your loved one's diagnosis for any other reason, you're certainly entitled to have the tests done a second time for additional confirmation. A second round of tests often is recommended, in fact, in questionable cases. You'll need to use a different diagnostic team, however, and because AD is progressive, it can be a good idea to wait 6 months to a year to see how results of the two rounds of tests compare. A noticeable decline in performances on the tests should be seen as additional evidence that AD may, in fact, be at hand.

Steps to the Truth

Here are the tests your loved one should expect. Not all of these tests may be ordered, as some cases of AD are easier to detect than others. If your loved one's condition is at all questionable, however, all of the following should be included for the diagnosis to be as accurate as possible.

Medical History

The purpose of this investigation is to get as much background as possible on the person's physical as well as mental health, including illnesses suffered in the past, illnesses that have been in the family, and how the person is now doing on a day-to-day basis. Ideally, it should be done in three stages: an interview with the person being evaluated alone, one with family members alone, and a third with the individual and family together.

Physical Exam

Not just Alzheimer's disease can cause memory lapses and mental confusion—more than 60 other conditions can, too—so the purpose of the physical exam is to look for signs that can help rule out these other possibilities. The person undergoing evaluation should expect routine inspections of things like blood pressure, pulse, and the appearance of the eyes and skin—possible indicators of problems such as nutritional deficiencies, thyroid problems, or troubles with the heart. The physical exam also will look for faulty connections within the nervous system, possible signs of problems such as brain tumors, Parkinson's disease, or stroke. To test for these conditions, the examiner will use procedures such as tapping on the knee with a hammer and pricking the skin to test for sensation—simple, but still valuable for assessing how well the body and brain are managing to stay in touch.

Laboratory Tests and Imaging Studies

These will include blood tests that look for bodily conditions such as infection, hormonal imbalances, and nutritional deficiencies, but they also may involve tests that look for problems that could exist in the brain. Often the brains of people with Alzheimer's disease will use less oxygen and glucose (blood sugar) than normal, or their brains may actually be smaller in an area known as the hippocampus due to brain cell destruction. Tests such as CT (computerized tomography) scans, PET (positron-emission tomography) scans, MRIs (magnetic resonance images), and EEGs (electroencephalograms) can help pick up these abnormalities. They also are good at finding evidence of other problems such as strokes, tumors, blood clots, and an accumulation of excess fluid within the brain's protective lining.

Evaluation of Mental Status

This part might be considered the "written portion" of the AD exam, requiring people under evaluation to respond to questions that test their ability to repeat simple phrases, do numeric calculations, and draw geometric figures. Because a person's occupation and level of education can influence performance on these tests, evaluators take these into consideration when scoring.

Psychiatric Evaluations

This series of tests takes the mental status exam to a higher level by using interviews and more written tests to assess a person's ability to communicate and reason. The psychiatric exam also can be helpful for determining the degree to which depression may be contributing to someone's mental decline.

The Mini–Mental Status Exam (MMSE) has been part of the standard repertoire for diagnosing AD since being introduced to the scientific community in the *Journal of Psychiatric Research* in 1975. The test appears simple, but it can be remarkably effective at detecting dementia. It works by assessing such functions as short-term memory, the ability to pay attention, language, and the capacity to follow written and spoken instructions. The MMSE includes questions such as "What day of the week is it?" and instructions to do simple tasks, such as remembering three objects named by the tester.[10] Because scores can be dependent on a person's age, occupation, and level of education, however, performances must be judged with these factors taken into consideration.

Depending on how the individual does on the MMSE, other tests may be given, including the Buschke Selective Reminding Test, which measures short-term verbal memory; the Wisconsin Card Sorting Test, which gauges the ability to deduce patterns; the Porteus Mazes test, which examines abstract puzzle-solving ability; and the Trail Making Test, which checks psychomotor skills by timing how long it takes for a person to connect consecutively numbered circles. Perhaps the simplest yet most informative test of all, however, is something called the Clock Test, which asks a person to draw the face of a clock on a blank piece of paper indicating a time specified by the instructor. Neurologists aren't sure why yet, but people suffering from some form of dementia will have trouble with this 90 percent of the time.

DISCLOSURE: WHOSE JOB IS IT?

When someone is tested for Alzheimer's disease, of course, there's always the chance of a "positive" outcome, and the subsequent difficulty of conveying this outcome to the person with the disease. How should news of a positive diagnosis be handled, and by whom?

"Almost" Alzheimer's: Mild Cognitive Impairment

As extensive as the diagnostic process for AD is, there still is a possibility that the verdict reached could be an inconclusive one that indicates not Alzheimer's disease but rather a recently identified, less severe form of memory loss known as *mild cognitive impairment* (MCI). Considered to be a kind of gray area between the benign forgetfulness commonly experienced by older people and the more problematic deficits characteristic of Alzheimer's disease, MCI still needs to be cause for concern because approximately 40 percent of people diagnosed with the condition will go on to develop AD within just 3 years.[11] Growing evidence indicates that MCI and Alzheimer's disease may share the same underlying biological processes, moreover, suggesting that MCI is not a separate condition but simply a form of AD in an earlier stage. Better methods of studying the brain while people with Alzheimer's are still living will need to be perfected, however, before this will be known for sure.

Many doctors in the AD field are now trained to handle this task, but families also are encouraged to assume the responsibility should they want to, says Daniel Kaufer, M.D., the director of clinical treatment at the Alzheimer's Research Center at the University of Pittsburgh. The normal procedure is for the family to be contacted when test results have been completed, and then be given the option of meeting with the doctor overseeing the diagnosis alone or with the person with Alzheimer's included, Dr. Kaufer says.

Which is preferable? "It's a judgment call," Dr. Kaufer says. "Sometimes families may want to attend this meeting without the patient, to have a chance to adjust emotionally to the news, while others will want the patient there, too, to hear the diagnosis firsthand."

However this meeting is handled, however, it's important that not too much ground be covered at once, Dr. Kaufer says. "The news in itself can be overwhelming, and families often will fail to make sense of treatment instructions that are offered at the same time. A follow-up meeting should be scheduled for discussing treatment and other necessary details when family members are in a less emotional state."

A recent survey by the Alzheimer's Association has shown the effects of this news-breaking session to be a considerable problem, in fact, as families commonly reported they had not received important treatment instructions at such meetings when in fact they had. The editors of the *Harvard Women's Health Watch* recently referred to this situation as a major "communication gap" between doctors and families of people with Alzheimer's, and the medical community has been hard at work to remedy it since.[12] "It's not uncommon for family members to be more traumatized by a diagnosis of AD than the patient," Dr. Kaufer says. "This is why it's important for this first meeting to deal with the diagnosis and the diagnosis only. Anything else that's covered probably just isn't going to sink in."

> *Families may want to attend this meeting without the patient, to have a chance to adjust emotionally to the news, while others will want the patient there, too, to hear the diagnosis first-hand.*
>
> —DANIEL KAUFER, M.D.

Tailoring the Truth

It's not hard to understand why a diagnosis of AD can be so difficult to accept, not just for the person with the illness but also for family members and friends. Here is a disease, after all, for which there is no known cure and that robs people of their memories, their ability to communicate, and eventually their minds. How is news of this magnitude best conveyed? Is honesty the best policy—to tell the whole truth and nothing but the truth, in black and white, with no room for deception motivated by compassion?

This is a difficult question, which most experts agree needs to be answered on an individual basis by each family, depending on the particular condition and temperament of the person who's been diagnosed. "If a person's condition is fairly advanced, full disclosure may not be necessary because the person might not fully comprehend it anyway," says Martin Diorio, Ph.D., a neuropsychologist who specializes in dementia diagnosis at the Good Shepherd Home in Allentown, Pennsylvania. "With people who still have adequate cognition, however, the truth becomes more important because they'll need to know why they'll be taking certain medications and undergoing other types of treatment."

People diagnosed with AD can find great value in taking part in support groups, visiting adult day care centers, and reading educational materials about their disease—none of which can happen, of course, unless the diagnosis is revealed. These individuals also may want to participate in any number of clinical trials now becoming available around the country that are testing new medications, nutritional remedies, hormonal treatments, as well as new diagnostic techniques. "Many people will have a desire to help science beat this disease," Dr. Diorio says, "but they can't do that, of course, unless their illness is disclosed."

The Patient's "Right to Know"

Another reason for disclosure has to do with our moral and even legal obligations to our loved ones, says Daniel Kuhn, M.S.W., the director of education at the Mather Institute on Aging. "A central principle of medical ethics is each person's 'right to know,' which states that everyone has a legal right to access the information contained in their medical records," he says. "Just as this provision allows patients the right to know the truth about cancer or any other illness where a diagnosis is required, it allows them the right to know the truth about Alzheimer's disease as well."

With this right to know can actually come a sense of relief when people learn the truth, Kuhn says. "They feel relieved that their symptoms can be attributed to a disease instead of something they have failed to control with willpower. It also allows them to discuss their difficulties openly instead of having to keep them hidden." Kuhn tells of one patient with AD, for example, who responded to his diagnosis with outright ease. "I knew something wasn't right," this man said, "so I worked hard for quite a while to cover it up. Perhaps now I don't have to be so careful if others know what's wrong with me."[13]

> *The walls of the prison we assume Alzheimer's to be may actually begin to break down for many people once the truth about their illness sets them "free."*

The walls of the prison we assume Alzheimer's to be, in other words, may actually begin to break down for many people once the truth about their illness sets them "free." By being aware of their condition, moreover, they can better understand not just their present circumstances but also what the future may bring. It helps to know the lay of the land, after all, before embarking on a difficult journey. By being prepared for the mental declines of AD in advance, Kuhn says, people with this illness may experience less torment and fear as it progresses.

THE DANGERS OF DENIAL

"Should I have known?" Eileen now asks herself. Her father had always seemed so self-sufficient, and although his memory had been slipping in recent years, Eileen assumed it was just par for the course for someone approaching 80. Besides, he seemed happy living with his younger sister, who had just retired and appeared to welcome the responsibility of overseeing his care.

But then Eileen received a phone call from her father's sister that he had run a stop light and caused a fairly serious car accident involving a mother and her two young daughters. "I felt horrible," Eileen recalls. "Should I have known? Should I have taken action sooner to have him tested and cared for at an appropriate facility? I guess I was in denial, but the truth just seemed too grim."

What motivates denial? In the case of Alzheimer's disease, it's fear. We hear the word *Alzheimer's* and see faces made of stone and bodies frozen in wheelchairs. "Our loved ones certainly can't have a disease that's going to do that," we say. David Shenk calls this kind of denial the "emotionally healthy choice" we make in response to situations "so horrifying that we need to pretend they do not exist."[14]

Be careful not to fall prey to the temporary shelter denial can provide. The truth about this disease must be faced sooner or later, and it's likely to be less painful when faced sooner.

FINDING "DR. RIGHT"

There's no question that AD is fast becoming one of our most pressing health problems and is only going to get more challenging as more of us succeed at extending our life span. Do not be surprised, however, if you're met with something less than enthusiasm when you consult with your loved one's doctor about overseeing your loved one's diagnosis. Research on AD, unfortunately, has run ahead of some physicians' confidence in treating it and also has outpaced the willingness of some health insurance companies to fund this treatment.

"All physicians are familiar with AD, but not all physicians are comfortable diagnosing it," says Daniel Kuhn. "Some see the lack of a single accurate test as an impediment, while others may shy from diagnosis because they feel unsure about how best to treat the disease." The medications available to treat AD, although effective in many cases, are new and without a proven track record, Kuhn explains, so some physicians simply may not feel confident about prescribing them.[15]

Some doctors also may be reluctant to get involved with treating AD because the process can require dealing with much more than just

Brenda and Norm: Fighting AD As a Team

"We first noticed a problem when we were vacationing in Europe and Norm started having trouble with the currency," says Brenda of her husband Norm, a Ph.D. in education diagnosed with AD 11 years ago at the age of 63. "Norm had always been so good with numbers, so it surprised us. Then when we got back home, Norm continued to have trouble with things like balancing the checkbook, paying the bill—things he usually could do in his sleep.

"Norm's very close with his doctor, so they got talking, and Norm agreed to undergo some tests to see what could be wrong, and that's when we discovered it was Alzheimer's. We were saddened by the news, of course, but the good part was that it gave us a focus

the person with Alzheimer's. A full understanding of the disease can demand consideration of so many factors—including the person's personality and dynamics within the family—that many primary care physicians, sadly, simply have trouble justifying the time, Kuhn says.

Don't be surprised, in other words, if even your own most venerable physician respectfully suggests you take your AD elsewhere. By no means should this advice discourage you from getting the best care possible for your loved one, however, because highly qualified doctors abound who are eager to deal with this most challenging disease. You just might not be able to find them at every local family medical center throughout the country.

If your loved one's doctor declines the task of overseeing the diagnoses and treatment of your loved one, ask him or her for the name of someone who might take the case. If he or she feels uncomfortable with even that, contact the local branch of the Alzheimer's Association in your area (see appendix) or your local medical society. Explain that you'd like to know how to get your loved one the most reliable diagnosis possible. More and more, hospitals, medical centers and special and something we could work against as a team. We agreed the very day we got the news that we were going to beat this thing as a team, and we've been working to do that ever since."

By seeking a diagnosis very shortly after Norm first started noticing symptoms—"maybe a year at most," Brenda says—Norm was able to begin a program of medications as well as physical and social activities that have had a remarkable impact on slowing the progression of his disease. "His doctors are amazed," Brenda says. "It's been almost 12 years since he was diagnosed, and he's still doing great. He has his good days and bad, of course, but we're still able to have dinner together and talk and maintain our relationship, and that's so important for both of us."

memory clinics throughout the country are making efforts to deal with the escalation of this disease.

THE SEVEN STAGES OF AD

Although no two cases of Alzheimer's disease will develop in the same way or at the same rate, researchers have been able to discern certain patterns in the progression of the disease that have allowed them to identify various stages. Not everyone with Alzheimer's will experience all of these stages to the same degree or for the same length of time. Some people may even skip certain stages entirely, so it's important to see these divisions as painting a very general picture of AD, at best. Alzheimer's can be as individual as the people who suffer from it, remember, a testimony to the complexity of the illness as well as the people it affects.

Stage 1. During this period, AD usually will show no outward symptoms at all, even though the process of nerve cell destruction and plaque accumulation has begun. It may take several years, in fact, before damage is sufficient for symptoms to appear.

Stage 2. The person will experience slight memory loss, often misplacing things or forgetting normally familiar names or events that have happened in the recent past.

Stage 3. Memory loss becomes more pronounced, often interfering with work and even making reading difficult as the person may not be

The "Second Childishness"

Writers and philosophers have been noticing the childlike behavior of people with Alzheimer's disease for centuries. "Old men are children twice over," wrote the Greek dramatist Aristophanes back in 419 B.C., a sentiment shared some 2,000 years later by Shakespeare, who called old age a time of "second childishness." Other noted figures throughout history also have noticed the parallel; for example, the Dutch scholar Erasmus wrote that the elderly seem to "grow backward into the likeness of children," and the personal physician of King Henry IV observed that old age is a time when "the senses . . . become as they were in unfancie [sic]."

Not until 1980, however, would this similarity be subjected to the scrutiny of modern science, and an amazingly accurate parallel it would prove to be. Thanks to the pioneering efforts of New York University neurologist Barry Reisberg, M.D., it's now become clear that AD progresses in stages that conform to the development of the human brain—only in reverse. The last abilities acquired are the first AD takes away, and the first functions mastered are the last AD rescinds. Memory, for example, which is one of the brain's later-acquired capacities, is among the first functions to be lost to Alzheimer's disease, while the capacity to smile, which is learned very early, is among the last.

Dr. Reisberg was able to observe this remarkable parallel not just by making comparisons of behavior but also by comparing brain able to remember what has been read just moments before. Routine trips to formerly familiar places may become problematic, along with remembering the names of everyday objects. Anxiety often will occur at this stage as a result of these impairments, accompanied by denial as a strategy of defense.

Stage 4. This stage may witness longer-term memory loss, such as forgetting social commitments or recent news events. Although denial

wave activity, glucose uptake by the brain, and tests of the nervous system. The closer Dr. Reisberg looked, in fact, the more the parallel seemed to hold true. It was as if AD was taking down, bit by bit, the tower of blocks that Mother Nature had worked so ingeniously over the years to construct.

Dr. Reisberg gave a fitting name to the phenomenon he discovered, calling it "retrogenesis," which means "back to birth." Further investigation would reveal the biological process behind it. Nerve cells within the brain can become active only when they develop a layer of insulation known as the *myelin sheath*—a coating required to keep brain signals from "shorting out" much as an electrical wire would if left bare. Scientists have found that AD first attacks this critical coating in areas of the brain that are the last to develop it—the hippocampus, for example, responsible for short-term memory. The last areas of the brain to succumb to AD, conversely, are those whose myelin sheath is constructed very early and are responsible for physical movement as well as such vital functions as the beating of the heart.[16]

The parallel also is one you might want to keep in mind when it comes time to deal with some of the more "infantile" behaviors AD can cause.

may still be prominent, the person may begin to withdraw from situations that cause difficulty, such as driving, doing household chores, or handling finances.

Stage 5. The person may now require help with activities of daily living, such as cooking and choosing appropriate clothing, although the ability to eat and use the bathroom may remain intact. Name recall also may now be a problem, especially names of grandchildren or siblings, and the ability to recall phone numbers and addresses will probably also be gone.

Stage 6. The person may now have trouble with even the most familiar names and usually will not be able to remember any recent events at all, although distant events may still be recalled. Help may be needed with even the most basic activities of daily life, such as bathing, eating, and using the bathroom. Delusional thinking and paranoia also may be a problem, possibly accompanied by violent behavior. Most people at this stage feel disoriented in time and place and may lack the ability to count even to 10.

Stage 7. At this stage the person usually is bedridden, incontinent, incapable of self-feeding, and unable to speak or communicate in all but the most rudimentary ways.

WHAT ELSE IT COULD BE

While Alzheimer's disease is the most common cause of dementia—responsible for over 50 percent of all dementias occurring in people older than 65—it is not the only one. More than 60 other medical conditions can cause mental impairments similar to those symptomatic of AD, the most common of which are listed here. Each of these possible causes needs to be ruled out before even a "probable" diagnosis of AD can be made, which is why the diagnostic process needs to be so extensive, but which is also why it's so important to have done: Approximately half of the conditions that can mimic Alzheimer's disease *can* be cured, and people tested for AD wind up having one of these conditions roughly 20 percent of the time. Pretty fair odds considering the alternative.

Vascular dementia. Formerly known as multi-infarct dementia (MID), this condition results from damage to brain tissue caused by multiple strokes (infarcts) due to impaired blood flow. Symptoms can include disorientation, confusion, disturbances in the ability to walk (including a history of falls) and changes in behavior. MID is neither reversible nor curable, but treatment of certain causative factors, such as high blood pressure, may help halt its progression.

> *Approximately half of the conditions that can mimic Alzheimer's disease can be cured, and people tested for AD wind up having one of these conditions roughly 20 percent of the time.*

Parkinson's disease. This disease affects control of muscular activity, resulting in tremors, stiffness, impaired speech, and eventually mental impairment, and it can coexist with AD in some people. Drugs have been developed that can help with the muscular problems caused by Parkinson's, but medications— even those used to treat AD—have so far been less successful at managing the mental aspects of the disease.

Depression. In addition to feelings of extreme sadness, hopelessness, physical fatigue, and thoughts of suicide, depression can mimic AD by causing memory loss and difficulty concentrating. Because depression becomes increasingly common with advancing age, moreover, it definitely needs to be ruled out before an accurate diagnosis of Alzheimer's disease can be made.

Huntington's disease. This is a hereditary disorder similar to AD in its symptoms of mental decline and changes in personality, but it can also include irregular movements of the facial muscles and limbs. The condition differs from AD in that it can be more clearly diagnosed.

Lewy body disease. Lewy body disease is a recently recognized condition characterized by symptoms resembling those of Parkinson's disease and AD combined. No treatment, unfortunately, yet exists.

Pick's disease. This is a rare brain disorder that affects an area of the brain known as the *frontal lobes* responsible for long-term memories and the ability to form logical thought. Shorter-term memory also can be harmed by Pick's disease in its early stages, however, in much the same ways as AD. The disease is also similar to AD in that it cannot be detected with certainty until a brain autopsy is done after death.

Normal pressure hydrocephalus (NPH). Often occurring in people who've had meningitis, encephalitis, or brain injury, NPH is a rare condition caused by an obstruction in the flow of spinal fluid. It can cause difficulty walking and incontinence in addition to impaired memory, but often it is correctable by surgery if diagnosed in time.

Creutzfeldt-Jakob disease (CJD). This is a rare, incurable, and fatal brain disease caused by infection, which can cause symptoms similar to those of Alzheimer's disease but which differs from AD by progressing very rapidly, usually causing death within a year.

Acquired immune deficiency syndrome (AIDS). AIDS can mimic symptoms of Alzheimer's disease when the virus responsible for the illness attacks nerve cells in the brain. The resulting impairments in mental function usually do not appear until the later stages of AIDS, however, after other serious illnesses also have begun to set in.

Other conditions capable of causing symptoms similar to those of AD include adverse reactions to certain prescription medications, liver and kidney problems, brain tumors, chronic alcoholism, blood clots in the brain, injuries to the brain, and late-stage syphilis. It's an extensive list, which is why diagnosing for AD needs to be such an extensive process. Not until all these conditions can be ruled out can Alzheimer's be ruled in.

A "WIN-WIN" FOR ALL

So what's to be gained by having a loved one tested for Alzheimer's disease? Quite simply everything—and for everyone concerned. Once a diagnosis is made, the person with AD can begin to benefit from a wide variety of treatments, as we'll be seeing in the chapter that follows, but family members and friends can begin to benefit, as well. "I was quite upset when I learned that my husband had Alzheimer's, of course," says Betty of her partner of over 40 years, "but in a way I was relieved, too, because it helped make sense of so much that hadn't been making any sense at all. Knowing that my husband has Alzheimer's also has taught me not to take his actions personally. I just tell myself that he has a disease, and that we both need to work together to manage it as best we can."

Let's take a look now at what this "management" of AD entails, first from the standpoint of medical treatment and then, in chapter 4, with respect to day-to-day care.

CHAPTER 3

Best Treatments from Modern Medicine— and Mother Nature, Too

❦

In the next 24 hours, another 1,000 people in the
United States will learn they have Alzheimer's disease, and
another 1,000 times the same question will be asked:
"What can be done about it, Doctor?"

UNTIL RECENTLY, THAT question didn't take very long to an-swer, because little could be done to help people with AD. But it's amazing what science can accomplish. Medications are now avail-able for treating Alzheimer's disease that might have been considered little more than wishful thinking as recently as 10 years ago, and huge strides have been made since then in treating the underlying causes of the illness, too. "It's an exciting time right now in Alzheimer's re-search," says Daniel Kaufer, M.D., the director of clinical treatment at the Alzheimer's Research Center at the University of Pittsburgh. "A lot of important discoveries are beginning to come together all at once and produce some very tangible results."

In the current excitement over pharmacological advances being made against AD, however, we mustn't forget the importance of supplementing these treatments with a "human" element. "These are not just people who need their neurotransmitters kept intact," says neuropsychologist Glenn Hammel, Ph.D., a consultant to the American Society on Aging who serves on the advisory board of Aegis Assisted Living. "They need help in keeping their identities intact, too, and that's our job as their caregivers, family members, and friends."

Consider yourself to be every bit as important in treating this disease as the latest drugs, in other words. "People with this illness need help staying in touch with themselves and the world around them, and we can do that by interacting with them in the right ways," says Paul Raia, Ph.D., the director of patient care for the Massachusetts chapter of the Alzheimer's Association in Cambridge. "People with Alzheimer's disease may lose the ability to initiate social interaction but not their need for it."

> *Consider yourself to be every bit as important in treating this disease as the latest drugs.*

Keep the importance of this "human" element in mind as we now take a look at the latest advances being made against AD by medical science. As we'll be explaining further in the next chapter, all of these treatments can be made more effective when supplemented by a safe and secure environment, stimulating activities, understanding, compassion, and love. Here's a brief summary of the treatments we'll be examining in this chapter:

1. Treatments for the cognitive symptoms of AD. These include newly developed medications that can help about half of all people with AD improve in such areas as memory, verbal skills, ability to concentrate, and facility with everyday tasks.

2. Treatments for the behavioral symptoms of AD. In this category are medications that, in conjunction with proper caregiving techniques, can help control the behavioral symptoms of AD such as agitation, physical aggression, depression, apathy, wandering, and delusional thoughts.

3. Treatments for the suspected causes of AD. These treatments encompass a variety of approaches ranging from anti-inflammatory medications and hormonal therapies to nutritional substances and compounds derived from herbs.

4. Treatments for the "person." Among these therapies are techniques such as music, aromatherapy, art, and massage, all of which can help people with Alzheimer's disease live with purpose and joy despite their cognitive declines.

Let's give this "four-wheeled" assault against AD a closer look.

TREATING THE COGNITIVE SYMPTOMS OF AD

As mentioned briefly already, scientists divide the symptoms of Alzheimer's disease into two basic categories. The *cognitive* symptoms of the illness include problems related to declines in mental acuity, such as memory loss, trouble forming coherent sentences, a need to repeat questions, difficulty concentrating, and trouble doing routine tasks. The *behavioral* symptoms of AD relate more to problems of mood such as feeling restless or agitated, being highly irritable, having bizarre notions, or acting withdrawn and depressed. Both types of symptoms can be treated, but different medications and methods are used. Let's look at how cognitive symptoms of AD are treated first.

Treating Cognitive Symptoms with Medication

Researchers got the idea for the cholinsterase inhibitors back in the late 1980s when it was discovered that people with AD have less of an important neurotransmitter in their brains, called *acetylcholine*, than people free of AD. If a medication could be developed that would make more acetylcholine available to keep nerve impulses flowing, researchers theorized, people with AD should be able to function better. These scientists soon found they were right. They developed a drug that helped preserve acetylcholine by inhibiting an enzyme (acetylcholinesterase) that causes acetylcholine to break down. The first of the cholinesterase inhibitors, as these medications have come to be called, is tacrine (Cognex). It was approved by the Food and Drug Administration (FDA) in 1993. Since then, three more cholinesterase inhibitors have gained FDA approval (see table 1), all of which work in the same basic way.

But how *well* do these drugs work, and what might be their side effects? Except for Cognex, which was found to be associated with liver damage and hence is now used only rarely, the most common side effects associated with the cholinesterase inhibitors are nausea, vomiting, diarrhea, and loss of appetite. These effects can vary widely from person to person, however, as can the effectiveness of these drugs, so don't be surprised if your loved one's doctor needs to try more than one cholinesterase inhibitor before the best and safest is found.

As for the effects of these drugs, most doctors agree they could be described as modest at best, yet this is a disease in which any improvement at all usually is much appreciated by both people with AD and their families. Improvements typically are in the areas of short-term memory, language skills, the ability to reason, and the ability to perform everyday tasks. It must be noted, however, that for as many as

Table 1. Cholinesterase Inhibitors

Generic Name	Brand Name	Year Approved
tacrine	Cognex	1993
donepezil	Aricept	1996
rivastigmine	Exelon	2000
galantamine	Reminyl	2001

one-half of people with AD, these medications may produce no noticeable improvements at all.[1]

Another drawback is that the medications appear to exert their
effects for a limited period of time—anywhere from a few months to
2 years, depending on the particular drug and the person's reaction to
it. By discontinuing these medications once they've been started,
moreover, most people with AD will experience a worsening of symptoms, so life-long use is recommended.

Turning Back the Clock?

Are these medications even worth it, you may be tempted to ask? The
answer will depend on your loved one's particular reaction, of course,
but according to Daniel Kuhn, M.S.W., the education director at the
Mather Institute on Aging, many families feel they are. "Family members report that the person with AD often seems sharper and more
attentive," Kuhn says. "The person's ability to recall recent events and
to complete personal care and household tasks
also may improve, and there may be noticeable
improvements in the person's mood as well as behaviors such as repeating questions, misplacing objects, or becoming confused in new surroundings.
Although the changes are seldom dramatic, the
families of those with AD are usually grateful."[2]

As for these drugs' ability to slow the development of the actual biological events thought to
cause Alzheimer's disease in the first place, "it's
still too early to say," reports Gary Small, M.D.,
the director of the Center on Aging and a professor of psychiatry and biobehavioral sciences at the
University of California at Los Angeles (UCLA). "We do know that
these drugs in some people can slow the progression of symptoms," he
says, "but we're less certain about the effects they might have on the
processes we believe to be responsible for these symptoms."

> As for the effects of these drugs, most doctors agree they could be described as modest at best, yet this is a disease in which any improvement at all usually is much appreciated by both people with AD and their families.

In the words of David Snowdon, Ph.D., a professor of neurology at the University of Kentucky Medical Center and the director of the much-publicized "Nun Study" of Alzheimer's disease being done at various convents throughout the United States, these drugs might be able to "shore up the river bank" against AD, but still to be determined is their ability to "stop the flood."[3]

Neither of these doctors' remarks should imply that the cholinesterase inhibitors can't be useful in helping people with AD and their families alike deal with this difficult disease, however. Time becomes precious in direct proportion to how much of it we have left, so the benefits of these drugs need to be judged accordingly. Even just a few more games of checkers or meaningful dinner conversations, for example, can be priceless if they're in danger of being among the last.

> *Time becomes precious in direct proportion to how much of it we have left, so the benefits of these drugs need to be judged accordingly.*

A Closer Look at the Cholinesterase Inhibitors

Which of these medications might be best for your loved one? It takes trying them to find out. According to Jeffrey Cummings, M.D., the director of the Alzheimer's Disease Center at the School of Medicine at UCLA, "One drug may be effective for one person but have side effects while that same drug for another person could be less effective but have no side effects." The goal, therefore, is to find which medications offer the most while sacrificing the least.

Tacrine (Cognex)

This was the first of the cholinesterase inhibitors, approved by the FDA in 1993 for people in the early and middle stages of AD, but clearly it is no longer the best. In addition to causing the same side effects as the other drugs in its class (including nausea, vomiting, diarrhea, and loss of appetite), Cognex may cause the additional problems of muscle pain, loss of coordination, rash, yellow skin or eyes, and changes in the color of the stools. Cognex also has been found to be ineffective in people with AD who carry a risk factor for the disease known as ApoE4, and it has to be taken several times a day. Clearly the most serious drawback to Cognex, however, has been its potential for caus- ing liver damage, a problem that requires its users to be tested weekly for over 4 months as a precaution.

*A*ricept is generally well tolerated and appears to be effective at reducing many of the symptoms of AD for periods ranging from 6 months to 2 years.

Understandably, Cognex is now the least used of the four drugs currently in the cholinesterase inhibitor class, but it does continue to be pre- scribed for people for whom it works and who are immune to its ill effects. A typical regimen is one pill four times daily in strengths that increase gradually over a period of several months.

Donepezil (Aricept)

Approved by the FDA in 1996, Aricept was the next drug to enter the battle against AD, and although it's no longer the newest, it does re- main the most widely prescribed. It's generally well tolerated and ap- pears to be effective at reducing many of the symptoms of AD for periods ranging from 6 months to 2 years. It was proven in one study to be superior to Cognex in improving cognitive function, and it en- joys the additional advantage over Cognex of working equally well in people with and without the ApoE4 gene.[4]

Aricept usually is given once a day as a 5-milligram tablet at around bedtime (or 2.5 milligrams if nausea is a problem), with an increase to 10 milligrams daily after 4 to 6 weeks if the drug is well tolerated. Side effects, in addition to the usual ones for the cholinesterase inhibitors, may include joint pain, sleeplessness, dizziness, drowsiness, or unusual dreams and are more likely with the heavier 10-milligram dose.

Rivastigmine (Exelon)

Approved by the FDA in April 2000, Exelon works in the same way as the other cholinesterase inhibitors, which is to help maintain levels of the important neurotransmitter acetylcholine in the brain. In its clinical trials, Exelon produced measurable improvements in mental functioning as well as activities of daily life and also helped improve or at least stabilize memory in about half the people with early to midstage AD who tried it for several months.[5] An advantage over Aricept and Cognex is that Exelon may be particularly effective against rapidly progressing AD, and it also may be superior to these other medications in treating later stages of the disease.

Exelon may be particularly effective against rapidly progressing AD, and it also may be superior in treating later stages of the disease.

Dosages usually begin at 1.5 milligrams daily with the goal being to increase this every 2 weeks until a final level of 6 to 12 milligrams is reached. Though side effects tend to be more common at these higher doses, they often can be reduced if Exelon is taken with meals. Available in both capsule and liquid form, Exelon also may increase the release of stomach acids in some people; hence, monitoring for stomach irritation may be necessary in people who suffer from stomach ulcers or who habitually use nonsteroidal anti-inflammatory drugs (NSAIDs), which also can irritate the stomach.

Galantamine (Reminyl)

Boasting an active ingredient derived from plants as common as the snowdrop and daffodil, this latest addition to the cholinesterase inhibitors was approved by the FDA in April 2001. Thus far, it appears to be the most promising of all. In one study done at Harvard University's Department of Psychiatry in Belmont, Massachusetts, 24 milligrams daily of Reminyl sharpened cognitive function, improved basic daily living tasks, and even delayed progression of behavioral symptoms—a collection of improvements that have researchers hoping this medication may have the best chance of treating the actual biological processes thought to be responsible for Alzheimer's disease.[6] While the most common side effects of Reminyl thus far have been the usual ones of nausea, vomiting, diarrhea, and decreased appetite, more time will be needed to see whether others emerge.

Available in tablets of 4, 8, or 12 milligrams to be taken twice daily, Reminyl given in doses of between 18 and 24 milligrams a day seems to have the greatest effects while still being well tolerated.

Which Drug Is Best?

Which of these drugs may be best for the person with AD in your life? Only your loved one's doctor, by trying these different medications, will be able to answer that question, so expect some experimentation until the best treatment is found. Know, too, that these medications stand their best chance of having a meaningful impact the earlier they're started in the course of the dis-

> *Researchers are hoping Reminyl may have the best chance of treating the actual biological processes thought to be responsible for Alzheimer's disease.*

ease—reason not to drag your feet any longer if you've been reluctant to have a loved one diagnosed. These drugs also can be effective in later stages of AD when behavior problems may begin to develop, however, so they needn't be ruled out just because early intervention may no longer be possible.

Natural Remedies for Cognitive Symptoms: Mother Nature Lends a Hand

The cholinesterase inhibitors mark a major breakthrough in the fight against AD, and even better ones should be coming soon, but the emergence of these medications shouldn't obscure the existence of other more "natural" treatments, some of which have been used successfully in other countries for many years. Don't be surprised, however, if none of these treatments is brought to your attention by your loved one's doctor. Because these treatments qualify as dietary supplements, they have not had to meet the strict approval standards of the FDA. Given the number of well-controlled scientific studies showing

Should You Try a Clinical Trial?

What if none of the currently available AD medications works for your loved one, or at least not well enough to justify the side effects or expense? Are you out of pharmacological options?

Not if you're willing to experiment. "If the antidementia treatments you have encountered prove disappointing, you may wish to enroll your loved one in a study of a newer, experimental one," says the education director of the Mather Institute on Aging, Daniel Kuhn, M.S.W. "The early stage of the disease is the proper time to consider this option, since people in later stages typically are excluded for a variety of medical, legal, and ethical reasons."[7]

While participation in such a study might seem risky, safety rarely is a problem, and the pros actually can outweigh the cons in many cases. "Participation in these studies involves no financial costs, and the risk of harm is minimal due to the ethical standards and strict protocols followed," Kuhn says.[8] If the drug turns out to be a success, of course, your loved one benefits by having access to a medication before it becomes available to the public. People participating in these trials often benefit from the intensive personal attention they get, too. Even if the drug they're given is an inactive placebo, which all well-controlled studies require, there can be positive outcomes from

the effectiveness of these treatments against AD, however, we feel obligated at least to make you aware of them as an option. As former USDA researcher and author of *The Green Pharmacy*, James Duke, Ph.D., says, "The drug companies and the FDA seem to be overlooking some promising herbal alternatives."[9]

Do keep in mind, though, that these are medicinally active substances that, although generally free of side effects, could react adversely with other medications your loved one may be taking. Get the approval of your loved one's doctor, therefore, before giving any of these treatments a try.

this treatment as well. Scientists call it the "placebo effect," and as a testimony to the power of hope, its results can be very real.

Know, too, that drug studies aren't the only type being conducted. Researchers also are studying better ways to diagnose AD, understand its risk factors, and manage it in ways that do not involve medications, and your loved one may also be able to join these types of studies. While there may be less chance for immediate personal benefit in these nonpharmacological studies, you and your loved one may still derive the satisfaction of knowing you're helping scientists in the AD battle. "People with AD and their families often feel good about their roles as volunteers in this important work, regardless of outcome," Kuhn says.[10]

For more information on how to enroll someone with AD in a clinical trial being conducted in your area, contact your local chapter of the Alzheimer's Association ([800] 272-3900), or check with the National Institute of Aging (NIA), which, in collaboration with the FDA, maintains a database of ongoing AD trials supported by both the federal government and private industry. The database is overseen by the NIA's Alzheimer's Disease and Education Referral Center (ADEAR), which can be called toll-free at (800) 438-4380 (Web site: www.alzheimers.org).

Huperzine-A

Derived from a rare type of club moss found in the cold climates of China, this over-the-counter dietary supplement is an updated version of a compound that has been used in traditional Chinese medicine for centuries. In a manner similar to the cholinesterase inhibitors, huperzine-A appears to aid mental function in people with AD by helping prevent the breakdown of acetylcholine, the important neurotransmitter that people with AD seem to lack. In one study of over 100 people with AD, 60 percent of those given huperzine-A for 8 weeks showed significant improvement in memory, thinking, and abilities to perform routine tasks.[11] Huperzine-A may even be able to boost brain function in people *without* AD, as suggested by another study that found the compound helped improve the memories of a group of students in middle school.[12] Huperzine-A may even help slow the progression of AD by reducing inflammation and helping prevent the buildup of amyloid plaques, says Alan Kozikowski, Ph.D., the director of the drug discovery program at the Georgetown Institute of Cognitive and Computational Sciences at the Georgetown University Medical Center in Washington, D.C.

In a manner similar to the cholinesterase inhibitors, huperzine-A appears to aid mental function in people with AD by helping prevent the breakdown of acetylcholine, the important neurotransmitter that people with AD seem to lack.

As for the safety of this herbal compound, no serious side effects have been reported, but avoidance by people with high blood pressure or severe liver or kidney disease is advised. Because neither the long-term safety of huperzine-A nor its interactions with other medications have been well studied, however, the substance should not be used without a doctor's approval. The recommended dosage for huperzine-A is 100 to 200 micrograms to be taken twice a day.

Ginkgo Biloba

Another herbal compound that's been doing some "heavy hitting" against Alzheimer's disease lately is an extract made from the leaves of the ginkgo tree known as *Ginkgo biloba*. Currently the most widely prescribed treatment for AD and other dementias in Germany, ginkgo is believed to work by stimulating nerve cell activity in the brain while also improving blood flow and perhaps protecting against further cell damage as an antioxidant.

The scientific evidence for ginkgo's impact against AD is substantial, including one study published in the much-respected *Journal of the American Medical Association* in 1997 in which people with Alzheimer's disease or other severe dementia showed significant improvement when given 40 milligrams of *Ginkgo biloba* extract three times daily for a year.[13] Not every study of ginkgo has produced such impressive results, but the evidence overall has been convincing enough for the herb to be recommended as a treatment for AD even by the normally conservative medical journal *The Lancet*, published in England. It also has piqued the interest of the National Institute on Aging (NIA) enough for it to allot $24 million for further study.

Note: The brain-boosting powers of ginkgo may not be limited just to people with AD or other dementias, as evidenced by one study in which 40 people between the ages of 55 and 86 with no cognitive impairment showed improvements in mental function after being given ginkgo for 6 weeks.[14] Other studies of people in their 20s and 30s, moreover, have suggested the herb may aid mental functioning regardless of age.[15]

Currently the most widely prescribed treatment for AD and other dementias in Germany, ginkgo is believed to work by stimulating nerve cell activity in the brain while also improving blood flow and perhaps protecting against further cell damage as an antioxidant.

Phosphatidylserine

The use of phosphatidylserine (PS) is another natural approach to treating Alzheimer's disease and other dementias that's been raising researchers' eyebrows lately, and for good reason. "The evidence for PS as a treatment for dementia is quite strong," reports Steven Bratman, M.D., the author of *The Alternative Medicine Sourcebook*.[16] Well-controlled studies involving over 1,000 people have found that phosphatidylserine—a compound once derived from the brains of cows but that more recently has been extracted from soybeans—appears to combat not just the mental declines associated with AD but depression as well. This was shown in one study of 494 elderly people with moderate to severe mental impairment who experienced significant improvement in mental functioning as well as depression after being given 300 milligrams of PS daily for 6 months.[17] PS has produced similar results in other studies of people with dementia, and the compound appears to help restore memory skills in older people without AD as well.[18]

Exactly how PS works to aid the brain is not fully understood, but it's believed to help brain cells maintain their basic structure in addition to serving as an essential building block of the chemicals that allow them to communicate with one another. PS appears to be quite safe, although concerns have been raised that it may interact unfavorably with heparin, a blood-thinning medication, and some experts worry that little is known of its long-term effects. The dosages that have been shown to be effective against AD and other dementias have ranged from 100 to 200 milligrams given twice daily.

Other Botanicals That Might Be Worth a Try

While the aforementioned substances technically are herbal, their degree of refinement separates them from the botanical remedies discussed next. Although their usefulness is considered questionable by most M.D.s, these herbs do come highly recommended by two widely respected leaders in the field of herbal medicine: David Winston, A.H.G., a widely respected herbalist and founder of Herbalist and Alchemist, Inc., in Washington, New Jersey, and James Duke, Ph.D., the author of *The Green Pharmacy*, who has studied medicinal plants everywhere from the jungles of the Amazon to the research labs of the USDA.

Is there any danger in trying more than one of these remedies at a time? Highly unlikely, Winston says. Certain herbal compounds are unwise to mix, but there are no known dangers to combining the antioxidant and circulation-stimulating properties of those discussed here. (Do get clearance from your loved one's doctor before trying any herbal compound, however, as some can interact adversely with prescription drugs.)

Rosemary. In addition to being a powerful antioxidant, rosemary contains compounds reported to help prevent the breakdown of the neurotransmitter acetylcholine in a manner similar to the cholinesterase inhibitors. The herb is best taken as a tea, but Dr. Duke suggests also adding it in the form of rosemary oil to bathwater or shampoos both to enjoy its soothing aromatic effects and to give it an opportunity to enter the bloodstream through the skin.

Gotu kola. This is another potent antioxidant and one that also can stimulate blood flow to the brain. It's available in capsules, tinctures, and creams.

Hawthorne. Yet another circulation booster with an antioxidant action, hawthorne has a long history in the treatment of heart disease but may be useful against Alzheimer's as well. It's available as an extract, capsules, or leaves for making tea.

St. John's wort. Best known for treating depression, this newsmaker also can be useful in helping repair nerve damage and thus may benefit people with AD. It's available in tincture and capsule form.

Bacopa. Not yet widely available in the United States, this is an herb that's been studied and used with great success in India. Like many of the other herbs useful against AD, it appears to increase blood flow to the brain. It's available in tincture form that can be added to beverages and foods.

Blueberries, strawberries, and spinach. Studies done with animals at the University of Colorado Health Sciences Center and Tufts University in Boston suggest these more edible botanicals also may help combat the ravages of AD.[19] They can be eaten in their natural state or, in the case of blueberries, as a spreadable extract that can give a whole new meaning to muffins or toast.

TREATING BEHAVIORAL SYMPTOMS OF AD

While the drugs for treating the cognitive symptoms of AD are relatively new, medications for treating the behavioral aspects of the disease have been in use for some time. These medications pose drawbacks, as

Brain Food by the Bowlful

Wait a second. An Alzheimer's remedy that can help soothe the soul as well as the synapses? Why not, says herbalist James Duke, Ph.D., who makes belly-warming, brain-stimulating soups with ingredients rich in choline, "a compound many researchers believe to be helpful for people with Alzheimer's disease," Dr. Duke explains. He seasons the soup with rosemary, sage, savory, and balm, which can "help the brain hold onto acetylcholine, another compound researchers believe to be helpful against this condition," he adds. Not all of these ingredients have to be used at once, Dr. Duke says, but do take note of them and try to use as many as possible to create brain-friendly meals:

- Barley
- Bottle gourd
- Dandelion flowers and greens
- Fava beans
- Flaxseed
- Lentils
- Poppy seeds
- Ground walnuts
- Cracked wheat

we'll be seeing shortly, but they can be virtual "sanity savers" for caregivers when all else has failed. "Caregivers mustn't be reluctant to allow the use of medications that can help make their loved ones more manageable," says Juergen Bludau, M.D., C.M.D., the medical director of the Morse Geriatric Center in West Palm Beach, Florida. "This illness can be difficult enough to manage without major behavioral problems to contend with."

It's important for caregivers to remember that every person will respond differently to these medications and that the medications may have side effects or react adversely with other medications the person may be taking. All of these possibilities should be discussed with your loved one's doctor before deciding to give any of these drugs a try.

Try TLC First

Before any medication is tried, the experts agree that efforts should be made to manage behavioral symptoms of AD in nonpharmacological ways first, which means with good old-fashioned "tender loving care." "The best nondrug treatment is a calm, well-rested caregiver who does not contradict or confront, who treats the patient with respect, and who inconspicuously fills in for the patient's deficits," says Myron Weiner, M.D., a professor of psychiatry at the University of Texas Southwestern Medical Center in Dallas.

We'll be going into this kind of personal care in far greater detail in chapter 4, but here's a quick overview to prepare you for what to expect. Efforts such as these can go a very long way— with or without the help of medications—to ease the burdens of this illness for all concerned.

> *Before any medication is tried, the experts agree that efforts should be made to manage behavioral symptoms of AD in nonpharmacological ways first, which means with good old-fashioned "tender loving care."*

The right environment. People with AD are easily affected by their surroundings, so you may need to make some changes to make sure your loved one is as comfortable as possible. Adequate lighting is absolutely essential for people with AD, and exposure to familiar personal possessions and memorabilia often can help them feel more secure and relaxed. Things to guard against are loud music, lots of hectic social activity, and generally anything that makes the person's world any more confusing than it already is.

Plenty of structure. Structure is critical for people with AD because they do best when they know what to expect. Predictability allows them to feel more at ease in a world that is getting less predictable all the time. You can help instill this sense of order by trying to help your loved one do things at the same time every day, such as dressing, bathing, eating, exercising, and engaging in recreational activities such as reading stories, painting, listening to music, dancing, or playing with a pet. The less uncertainty in the life of people with

Alzheimer's, the better they generally will feel, and the less difficult their behavior is apt to be.

Treating Behavioral Symptoms with Medication

If caregiving efforts fail to keep difficult behaviors under control, it may be necessary to talk to your loved one's doctor about the advisability of using a medication. Many are now available, each with a specific action designed to help control particular types of behavior problems.

Treating Depression

Depression is common in people with AD for psychological as well as biological reasons. People with the illness often feel understandably saddened to have such a tragic disease, but they also can feel depressed about being a burden to their families, or they may worry about being abandoned, or they may feel a growing sense of alienation due to their waning mental skills. Add AD's tendency to reduce levels of the mood-elevating neurotransmitter serotonin in the brain, and it becomes clear why depression among people with AD is so widespread.

Fortunately many medications are now available for treating depression in people with AD, however, the most common being in a class known as *selective serotonin reuptake inhibitors* (SSRIs). Dr. Weiner, for example, usually prescribes one of the SSRIs for his AD patients, "namely Prozac, Zoloft, Paxil, or Celexa, usually in about half the regular adult dose," he says. "Prozac is long acting, so it can be given as infrequently as once a week. The others should be given once a day in the morning, because they may interfere with sleep." Other antidepressants currently being used to treat depression as well as other depression-related disorders in people with AD, such as anxiety, include the following:

- Bupropion (Wellbutrin)
- Desipramine (Norpramin or Pertofrane)
- Fluvoxamine (Luvox)

- Nefazodone (Serzone)

- Nortiptyline (Pamelor or Aventyl)

- Trazodone (Desyrel)

Treating Apathy

Apathy often is confused with depression in people with AD, but it's a separate problem and is actually more common in people with AD than depression. It's characterized by a lack of emotion and enthusiasm for life in general and may be accompanied by sadness, frequent crying, and feelings of hopelessness. People with AD who suffer from apathy usually respond better to stimulants such as methylphenidate (Ritalin) than they do to antidepressants, so be sure your loved one's doctor considers the possibility that apathy rather than depression could be your loved one's problem. Be forewarned, too, that it can be one of the more difficult AD behaviors to treat.

Treating Symptoms of Psychosis

Symptoms of psychosis can be among the most difficult for caregivers to manage because they can be quite physical in nature, including physical aggression, wandering, strange reactions to hallucinations, and extreme irritability. Fortunately, these behaviors usually can be treated with the right medication, including the ones listed here:

- Carbamazepine (Tegretol)

- Divalproex (Depakote)

- Haloperidol (Haldol)

- Olanzapine (Zyprexa)

- Risperidone (Risperdal)

Treating Sleep Problems

Sleep problems are common in people with AD, but sleep medications must be used carefully because many can reduce coordination and increase the risk of falls. "For sleep problems associated with AD, I use trazodone (Desyrel) in doses from 25 to 200 milligrams at bedtime," says Dr. Weiner. Some studies suggest that daytime exposure to bright light can be another way to help people with AD sleep better,[20] and, as we'll be seeing in chapter 4, daily exercise also can help.

Treating Agitation

Most people with AD, 70 to 90 percent, experience agitation at some point, often as a result of their general state of confusion made worse by their difficulty in expressing it. Agitation also may be a sign that the person with AD is experiencing some sort of physical discomfort, such as an infection, so it's important to rule out these possibilities before assuming that all you're dealing with is a problem of mood.

Many drugs are available for treating agitation, but caregivers should know that it often will resolve itself if they can be patient and create a soothing environment.

Many drugs are available for treating agitation, but caregivers should know that it often will resolve itself if they can be patient and create a soothing environment. This outcome was observed in one study that found that people with AD in an assisted living facility showed similar reductions in agitation over 4 months whether they were medicated or not.[21] Because many drugs used to treat agitation can have unwanted side effects such as mental confusion, dizziness, drowsiness, and slurred speech, they should be used only as a last resort. Here are some of those available now:

- Alprazolam (Xanax)
- Buspirone (Buspar)
- Citalopram (Celexa)
- Diazepam (Valium)
- Fluoxetine (Prozac)
- Lorazepam (Ativan)
- Paroxetine (Paxil)
- Sertraline (Zoloft)[22]

TREATING THE SUSPECTED CAUSES OF AD

So far, we've looked at the methods scientists now have for treating both the cognitive and behavioral symptoms of Alzheimer's disease. It's time now to examine the progress that's being made in treating the actual *causes* of AD. As can be seen from the following sections, the gamut of treatments being used in the battle against AD is a wide one—proof of just how committed scientists are to getting control of this potentially devastating disease.

Anti-Inflammatory Medications

It might seem like a case of David against Goliath—that drugs as common as aspirin and ibuprofen could have an impact against such a medical monster as Alzheimer's disease—but this is what research suggests. To understand why, let's take a quick look at a case of Alzheimer's disease in progress.

In response to damage being done to brain tissue by Alzheimer's disease, the body rushes an emergency crew of compounds called *prostaglandins* to the site of injury with hopes of stopping the damage and beginning a process of repair. But a little like that plumber who ruins the carpet with muddy shoes, these prostaglandins sometimes can do more harm than good, exacerbating rather than ameliorating the problem. Scientists noted this result when studies started showing that medications known to reduce inflammation in the body also seemed to reduce risks of Alzheimer's disease.

In one such study, completed in 1996, people who regularly used anti-inflammatory medications (such as aspirin, ibuprofen, and naproxen sodium, as well as prescription drugs commonly used for arthritis) were found to be 30 to 60 percent less likely to develop AD than people who did not use these medications.[23] In an earlier study that compared identical twins, researchers found that people who had habitually used anti-inflammatory medications for arthritis were 10 times less likely to develop AD than their siblings who had not.[24] In studies with mice genetically engineered to develop AD, moreover, researchers have found that anti-inflammatory compounds can limit the formation of amyloid plaques already in progress.[25]

As a result of these studies, some doctors treating people with AD now prescribe anti-inflammatory medications on what's known as an "off-label" basis. William Markesbery, M.D., the director of neurology at the Sanders-Brown Center on Aging at the University of Kentucky Medical Center, along with David Snowdon, Ph.D., has been analyzing the data gathered as part of the much-publicized Nun Study dedicated to unraveling the mysteries of Alzheimer's disease. Dr. Markesbery recommends that his Alzheimer's patients take a prescription anti-inflammatory medication such as Celebrex, in addition to higher-than-normal amounts of vitamin E, vitamin C, and folic acid. Common over-the-counter anti-inflammatory drugs such as aspirin, ibuprofen, and naproxen sodium are known to have similar anti-inflammatory properties as the prescription anti-inflammatories, but they are more prone to cause stomach irritation, Dr. Markesbery reasons.[26]

> *Some doctors treating people with AD now prescribe anti-inflammatory medications on what's known as an "off-label" basis.*

Note: Celebrex belongs to a relatively new class of anti-inflammatory drugs known as COX-2 inhibitors that reduce inflammation by inhibiting the formation of prostaglandins—those "plumbers with the muddy shoes" mentioned earlier. Others in this class of drugs that are commonly used to treat arthritis are rofecoxib (Vioxx) and meloxicam (Mobic). While their effects against AD may look promising, most doctors agree that it's premature to be using them to treat AD until further testing has been done. Long-term use may cause stomach problems as well as difficulties with the kidneys and liver.

Estrogen: Protection for Women

This perennial newsmaker first had its hat pulled into the AD ring in 1993 when scientists found that women who had been undergoing estrogen replacement therapy (ERT) after menopause had lower rates of AD than women who had not been receiving the hormone. The results of subsequent research added further evidence. Depending on how much of the hormone had been given and for how long, estrogen replacement therapy seemed to reduce a woman's chances of getting AD by between 40 and 70 percent.[27]

The reasons for this protective effect? Scientists aren't sure yet, but they have identified some possibilities:

- Estrogen may trigger the growth of nerve pathways involved with memory.

- Estrogen seems to increase blood flow to the brain by smoothing, relaxing, and opening blood vessels.

- Estrogen may slow or stop the production or action of beta-amyloid, the protein that causes the harmful plaques associated with AD.

- Estrogen may help reduce the inflammation associated with beta-amyloid and other proteins in the brain.

- Estrogen seems to stimulate production of depleted neurotransmitters, such as acetylcholine and serotonin, so important for normal functioning of the brain.

- Estrogen has antioxidant properties, which could help control the production of free radicals thought to contribute to AD.

While estrogen may help protect against AD, however, scientists have not yet been able to prove it can help treat existing cases of the disease.

While estrogen may help protect against AD, however, scientists have not yet been able to prove it can help treat existing cases of the disease. In two well-controlled studies, women with Alzheimer's disease were given estrogen but showed no discernible changes in decline. Researchers speculate that once the illness has taken root and done considerable damage, estrogen may in a sense be "out of its league" in being able to alter the process to any appreciable degree. In both of the studies mentioned, for example, the women given estrogen had been suffering from AD for some time.[28]

Treatment of existing cases aside, scientists still are hard at work to further understand estrogen's protective effects. One study, sponsored by the National Institutes of Health and scheduled for completion in 2002, is following 7,600 healthy postmenopausal women in hopes of determining the degree to which estrogen may help protect women from AD even when started late in life. An offshoot of this study, called the Women's Health Initiative Study of Cognitive Aging, will attempt to determine whether estrogen might be protective against the declines in memory that tend to be associated with the aging process in general. In other words, we still have much to learn about estrogen's role in the Alzheimer's story.

Might estrogen be protective against AD in men? Unfortunately, such use in men runs the risk of causing unwanted side effects that might outweigh the benefits, researchers say.

Antioxidants: Free Radicals Under Arrest

While the cholinesterase inhibitors represent the best treatment modern science has been able to develop to slow the progress of AD so far, another approach that has researchers excited hasn't had to stray as far from the ways of Mother Nature. Nutritional compounds called *antioxidants* are showing promise against AD, and a quick tour inside the brain will help show why.

Brain metabolism requires the use of lots of oxygen, a process known as *oxidation*, but an unfortunate side effect of this process is the production of molecular troublemakers called *free radicals*. Because these molecular malcontents lack an electron to keep them chemically stable, they go around stealing electrons from other molecules, thus weakening the cells these molecules comprise (see figure 3.1). Cells ravaged by free radicals cannot function as they should, the result

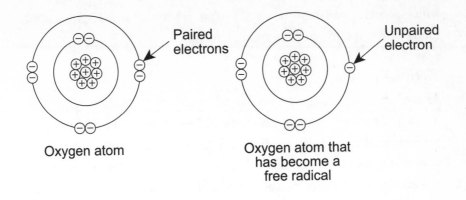

Paired electrons

Unpaired electron

Oxygen atom

Oxygen atom that has become a free radical

Figure 3.1—*Free Radicals*

being health problems that can range from facial wrinkles to heart disease, depending on the type of cells that have been harmed.

What if these cells under attack happen to be nerve cells in the brain? Double trouble, scientists fear, because in addition to having a high metabolism (and hence high rate of free-radical production), brain cells tend to have a low stockpile of antioxidants on hand for protection. Worse yet, research suggests that when brain cells begin to suffer damage from AD, free-radical production is driven even higher, perhaps as a result of increased metabolic activity created by immune cells trying to defend against the damage. The result can be added injury as the body's attempts at repair could make the damage even worse.

Antioxidants to the rescue. By sacrificing electrons of their own, these molecular heroes help deactivate free radicals and thus help protect cells throughout the entire body from harm—brain cells included. Our bodies produce some antioxidants as part of normal metabolism, but these supplies sometimes can become outnumbered,

> *Cells ravaged by free radicals cannot function as they should, the result being health problems that can range from facial wrinkles to heart disease, depending on the type of cells that have been harmed.*

which points to the importance of getting additional antioxidants in the foods we eat and in nutritional supplements.

Victories for Vitamin E

As we'll be explaining in more detail in chapter 7, a diet rich in antioxidants, as well as other key nutrients, may be one of the strongest defenses against AD that we can mount. Better yet, it may be a way to slow down cases of Alzheimer's disease already in progress. This point was shown in a landmark study reported in the prestigious *New England Journal of Medicine* in 1997 in which people with AD who were given high doses of vitamin E (or another antioxidant, selegiline) experienced a slowdown in the development of many of their symptoms by about 7 months. The group given the antioxidants also lived longer, were able to stay out of nursing homes longer, and were not as quick to lose their abilities to do everyday tasks as a similar group not given the antioxidant advantage.[29]

Scientists also are looking into the possible value of combining vitamin E with the cholinesterase inhibitor donepezil (Aricept), as witnessed by a study currently in progress by the National Institutes of Health called the Memory Impairment Study. Seven hundred people with memory problems (but not clinically diagnosed Alzheimer's disease) are being given a combination of Aricept and vitamin E for 3 years to see whether fewer might develop AD than statistics would predict.[30]

Benefits from Other Antioxidants

Might other antioxidant nutrients also have a favorable impact against Alzheimer's disease? Researchers are beginning to think so, and several large-scale studies are currently underway to help shed further light. Besides vitamins E and C, flavonoids (compounds prevalent in many fruits, vegetables, and herbs) are rich sources of antioxidants, as are vitamin B_{12}, folic acid, and the herb *Ginkgo biloba*, to name just a few. Certain foods also are uniquely potent sources such as blueberries, strawberries, spinach, and other leafy green vegetables (as we'll be seeing in chapter 7), so these shouldn't be overlooked, either.

But while getting antioxidants in foods is one thing, should we for any reason be wary of upping the ante and exceeding currently recommended levels by taking supplements? The answer depends on the nutrient, of course, and also what medications a person might be taking, but most experts currently involved in the treatment of Alzheimer's disease see more benefit than harm in going the supplement route—within reason, of course, and under a doctor's supervision only. Roger Rosenberg, M.D., a professor of neurology at the University of Texas Southwestern Medical Center,

> *Most experts see more benefit than harm to going the supplemental route—within reason.*

recommends his patients with AD take as much as 2,000 IU of vitamin E daily—the amount shown to be effective in the 1997 study reported in the *New England Journal of Medicine*. Other doctors are more conservative, advising 400 IU twice daily. This amount is "safe for most individuals and should have the antioxidant effect desired in the brain," says John C. Morris, a professor of neurology at Washington University at St. Louis.

Anyone taking vitamin E—or any supplement, for that matter—should discuss the matter first with their physician, however, because adverse reactions with other medications—warfarin (Coumadin), for example—can occur.

TREATING THE "PERSON"

As impressive and encouraging as the recent medical developments against AD have been, there's not a single one that can't work even better when used along with treatments that take a more basic approach and help the person with AD help him- or herself. "As people with this illness begin to lose their higher thought processes, it becomes increasingly important for them to be kept in touch with the

Beware of the Bogus

By its very nature, Alzheimer's disease welcomes exploitation. The compromised mental capacities of those who have the illness, combined with the desperation often felt by their caregivers, can lead to bad decisions being made about bad products, with bad results. How to spot a sham?

"Basically, the old adage holds true that if something sounds too good to be true, it probably is," says Glenn Hammel, Ph.D., a neuropsychologist and consultant to the American Society of Aging, who specializes in helping protect the legal rights of people with Alzheimer's disease and other dementias. Consider, too, that if the world's top scientists haven't yet been able to develop dramatically effective treatments for Alzheimer's disease, why should we trust that any lesser experts might?

world through their more basic senses, such as sight, sound, smell, and touch," says Paul Raia, Ph.D., the director of patient care for the Massachusetts chapter of the Alzheimer's Association in Cambridge. "Research shows that people with Alzheimer's disease who are kept stimulated in these ways not only are happier and have fewer behavior problems but often experience a slowdown in the progression of their disease."

In testimony to the importance of keeping people with AD stimulated, Dr. Raia has developed a program he calls "Mental Floss" (discussed later), which seeks to keep people mentally and physically active a full 8 to 10 hours a day. "The use-it-or-lose-it approach that's important for maintaining mental acuity in all of us is no less important for people with AD, and it may be even more important given the disease process they're up against," he says. "It's a great tragedy to assume that no harm is done by letting people with this illness sit idle."

As we'll be seeing in more detail in chapter 7, researchers are beginning to suspect that mental activity may help spur new neurological connections in the brain in much the same way as physical exercise can spur the growth of new blood vessels in the muscles and heart. The brain that stays mentally active, therefore, may quite literally learn ways to "get around" the damage AD begins to cause.

Preserving the Present by Way of the Past

What kind of activities might be appropriate as part of a comprehensive "mental flossing" program? "That's different for every person, of course," Dr. Raia says, "but basically you want to encourage activities and interests that have been a part of the person's past." Any new activity, caregivers need to remember, is only going to frustrate the person with AD because they have lost the ability to learn, he adds.

This doesn't mean that skills already established can't be keep alive and quite well, however. Herein lies another aspect of the caregiver's challenge: to find what past interests still can excite, to excavate old memories that still may bring a sense of purpose and joy. Because AD by its very nature prevents the development of anything new, we need to dig inside the person with AD and make the most of what's left of the old.

Because AD by its very nature prevents the development of anything new, we need to dig inside the person with AD and make the most of what's left of the old.

Consider the following therapies with that goal in mind. Yes, we need to help the person with AD cope with the present, but, as we'll see, cultivating interests of the past often can help do just that.

Music: Communication You Can Dance To

When William Congreve remarked in 1697 that "Music hath charms to soothe a savage breast, / To soften rocks, or bend a knotted oak," he might have been talking about the power of this unique art form to touch the hearts and minds of people with Alzheimer's disease. "The part of the brain that governs the ability to appreciate music is one of the last areas to be affected by Alzheimer's disease, which explains why [people with AD] often will respond to music even in later stages of their disease," says Dr. Raia. He tells the story of one caregiver who learned to get his wife through her most cranky "sundowning" periods late in the afternoon by putting on old Glenn Miller records. "The two would dance for 45 minutes to an hour, and she'd be a whole new person afterward," he says.

Music's therapeutic benefits for people with AD have been well documented in scientific studies reported over the past decade in the *Journal of Music Therapy*. Appetite stimulation, decreased wandering, better sleep, fewer problems with bathing, improved language skills, and increased willingness to socialize—all have been shown to be among the "magic" music can work. "Of all forms of communication," Dr. Raia says, "music seems to be the most universal."

> *Appetite stimulation, decreased wandering, better sleep, fewer problems with bathing, improved language skills, and increased willingness to socialize—all have been shown to be among the "magic" music can work.*

How can music be used best? "Try to find what the person likes," suggests Michelle Ritholz, a certified music therapist at the Nordoff-Robbins Music Therapy Center in New York. "Often it will be music the person has been familiar with in the past, but don't be afraid to try a variety of styles." And don't assume that just because a song is happy and upbeat that it will always produce a positive response. "If a person is acting depressed, sometimes it can be better to match their mood with something fairly somber at first, playing happier songs gradually to coax rather than coerce them into a more positive state of mind," says Ritholz.

Art: Pictures Worth a Thousand Words

When the world-famous painter Willem de Kooning discovered he had Alzheimer's disease in the late 1970s, he feared his art would suffer as much as his brain. But it did not. Despite severe memory loss, speech problems, and even physical disabilities, de Kooning went on to produce works valued by some critics as the best of his career. "Collectively, the pictures . . . seem to glow with an inner light," art critic David Bonetti of the *San Francisco Examiner* wrote of de Kooning's later works. "They remind you that even during bleak times, art can offer emotional and spiritual solace like nothing else."[31]

Neurologist Hogo Espinel expressed a similar view in an essay in the British medical journal *The Lancet*. "These paintings are not merely the product of someone who had simply retained colour perception and the motor strength to copy. Even if he at times confused his wife with his sister . . . de Kooning went on to create. His resurgence is a testimony to the potential of the human mind, evidence for hope."[32] The curator of the San Francisco Museum of Modern Art, Gary Garrels, went so far as to tell art journalist Kay Larson that the works from de Kooning's Alzheimer's years "are among the most beautiful, sensual, and exuberant abstract works by any modern painter."[33]

Indeed, even though many other aspects of his intellect were shutting down, de Kooning's emotional centers were not, and he retained the ability to express these emotions through the paints of his palette and the bristles of his brush. "Art is a language unto itself, helping us to say things we don't have words for," says Nancy Gerber, M.S., director of the graduate school of art therapy education at M.C.P. Hahnemann University in Philadelphia. And herein lies its value for people with Alzheimer's disease. Art therapist Laura Greenstone, a consultant with Creative Arts Therapy Resources in Philadelphia, tells the story of Albert, who even in the advanced stages of AD was able to progress from painting just circles to painting highly recognizable forms. "We had tapped into a deep piece of his self-esteem," she says. "The process of creating art had stimulated a cognitive function in his brain, and even though he never became verbal,

> *Art isn't limited to reawakening just emotional states. It also can help people with AD "brush up" on the hand–eye coordination needed for tasks such as eating and dressing.*

his attention span improved, he was less agitated, and he was better able to calm himself down. He used art to become more connected to the world."

But art isn't limited to reawakening just emotional states. Greenstone says it also can help people with AD "brush up" on the hand–eye coordination needed for tasks such as eating and dressing. Not bad for a therapy that could make for some interesting decoration, too.

Massage: Instant Intimacy

Massage may seem more fitting for people with ailing muscles than ailing minds, but many massage therapists report the power of touch can work wonders for people with AD and other dementias and for a reason that may be as simple as touch itself. "No other form of communication is as direct," says Dr. Raia. "There's a simplicity and unencumbered intimacy in the power of touch that seems to resonate especially well in people affected by this disease." Dr. Raia says that in addition to helping a person with AD physically by improving circulation and loosening tight muscles, massage can have a long list of psychological benefits such as reducing anxiety, aiding sleep, reducing the need for sedating medications, controlling problem behaviors, and helping orient the person in both time and space.

> *In addition to helping a person with AD physically, massage can have a long list of psychological benefits.*

It's important when giving a massage to someone with AD, however, to dispense with many popular notions of what a massage should be, says Dawn Nelson, the founder and director of Compassionate Touch for Those in Later Life Stages. No slapping or karate chops, please. You may need to be quite careful, in fact, not to frighten or in any way threaten the person in your initial approach. Start by explaining as simply and gently as possible what you would like to do, perhaps holding the person's hand or lightly touching a shoulder as first points of contact. After that, "work slowly and sensitively, with nonjudgmental hands," Nelson says. The important thing is to make contact with the person one-to-one on an "intuitive level," she says, being "creative, flexible, patient, and adaptable, doing whatever seems to work. Nothing should be forced, not even the length of the massage," she adds. Finally, if the person doesn't seem receptive one day, accept that reaction, but do offer a massage again another time.

Totally forget the rough stuff, in other words. You're trying to express with your hands the love and compassion that you feel in your heart but that words may no longer be able to convey. Do it right, and you stand a good chance of getting through to the person with Alzheimer's disease "in ways nothing else can," Nelson says.

Aromatherapy

Although the practice has been around since biblical times, aromatherapy gained its first practitioner of the modern era somewhat by accident in 1920. While working in a perfume factory, French chemist René-Maurice Gattefossé suffered a severe burn and was amazed at how quickly it healed when he applied some lavender oil he happened to have on hand. Since then, aromatherapy has gone on to be a legitimate healing modality—and one with definite benefits for people with Alzheimer's, says aromatherapist Diane Grandstrom, R.N., B.S.N., C.C.R.N. "People with this illness know something isn't right, and it causes them a tremendous amount of anxiety," Grandstrom says.

Scents to the rescue. Certain aromas generated by essential oils can do a lot to help dispel the angst associated with AD—sweet orange, especially, Grandstrom says. "Lavender is another calming scent, but most people find the fragrance of sweet orange more pleasing." To impart this calming pleasure, all that's needed is some essential oil of sweet orange—"Look for 100 percent pure," Grandstrom suggests—plus some distilled water and a small squirt bottle known as a mister, all available at minimal cost at most health food stores. Simply add the oil a drop at a time to about 2 ounces of water until the strength of the fragrance "seems right," which will usually be about 10 drops, Grandstrom says. And don't be afraid to try "cocktails," she adds. Lavender and sweet orange together can make an especially relaxing combination—for caregivers, too.

How to dispel these calming aromas? Use the mister to spritz above your loved one's head, or spritz and let him or her walk into the

---

"Mental Floss"—Clearing New Neural Pathways

When Paul Raia encourages people with AD to sing, dance, play word games, do art projects, and reminisce about the good old days, he's not just helping them kill time. He's helping them create new neurological connections in their brains. Based on laboratory experiments with mice showing that previously underutilized areas of the brain can be encouraged to form new neurological pathways when stimulated by certain activities, Dr. Raia has put together a series of exercises designed to do essentially the same thing in people with AD, thus helping "bypass" the damage done by their disease. "With these activities, we try to create a cross modal transfer where information is transferred to other parts of the brain so it can be preserved for a longer period of time," Dr. Raia explains.

In addition to improving cognitive skills, these activities can help people with AD avoid negative moods and be more sociable, Dr. Raia says. "People with Alzheimer's disease may lose their ability to initiate social interactions, but not their need for it."

Some of the activities Dr. Raia recommends are described here. These activities should never be forced on a person, he stresses, but rather only offered. Remember, too, that the purpose of these activities is to entertain, not exasperate. If at any point your loved one appears frustrated, stop and try something simpler. Also avoid the temptation to be overly patronizing by treating your loved one in a childish manner when working at these exercises, Dr. Raia says.

mist, whichever approach seems preferred, Grandstrom says. You also can let your loved one simply sniff from the misting bottle throughout the day as often as desired. Another way to use essential oils is to add them to bathwater to make bathing a less traumatic experience for people with AD, says Frena Gray-Davidson, the director of Self-Help Alzheimer's Caregiver's Training and Information (SHACTI).[34]

Many people with AD easily take offense at feeling demeaned in this way, so it's important to work at these exercises in ways that show sensitivity and respect. Here are some exercises to try:

- Read a paragraph from a book, and ask the person with AD to summarize its main ideas.

- Place about a half a dozen familiar objects in a bag (such as a flashlight, spoon, pencil, pair of eyeglasses) and ask your loved one, with eyes closed, to identify each object by touch.

- Ask your loved one to clap or tap on something in time to a rhythmic piece of music.

- Ask the person with AD to read something, writing down every 10th word.

- Ask your loved one to draw a basic floor plan of your house.

- Present the person with drawings of ten clocks with numbers but no hands, and ask him or her to draw the missing hands to indicate times that you specify.

- Get together some modeling clay and ask your loved one to form various familiar shapes, such as a car or house, or more basic ones, such as a circle, triangle, or square.

- Infuse cotton balls with various scents, put them into small bottles, and ask the person with AD to try to distinguish among them, identifying the scents if possible.

But will these scents work for people with AD who have lost their normal ability to smell? Davidson says essential oils have the power to work on the brain directly and hence do not need to be recognized in order to produce a relaxing effect.[35]

NO STONE UNTURNED

As you can see, the medical community is leaving no stone unturned in its efforts to make life better for people with Alzheimer's disease. While medications are being perfected to retard the progression of this illness from a biological standpoint, AD's symptoms are also being attacked in more personal ways through activities such as music, art, and dance.

As we'll be seeing in chapter 4, however, the greatest treatment responsibilities often lie not with trained professionals, but rather with people like you, the family members or friends who take care of the person with AD on a daily basis.

CHAPTER 4

Caregiving:
A Crash Course

❧

*The presence or absence of caring people may be
the most significant factor in determining the
quality of life for someone with AD.*

—DANIEL KUHN, M.S.W., DIRECTOR OF EDUCATION
AT THE MATHER INSTITUTE ON AGING

As doctors are doing their best to treat Alzheimer's disease with
their medicines, millions of Americans are doing their best to
treat it in a different, perhaps even more important way. They're
brushing teeth, zipping zippers, and combing hair. They're reading
stories, taking walks, washing clothes, and drying tears. We're talking
about people like you—the caregivers who constitute the closest thing
to a cure for AD that we currently have. Until we can learn more
about how to stop the causes of this disease, we're going to have to do
our best to manage the symptoms, and good caregiving is the best way
to do just that.

Good caregiving is a tremendous challenge, but it's also one that
can be met, and in this chapter we'll see how. We'll start by taking a

101

look at the world as someone with Alzheimer's disease might see it, to help you get a better understanding of the behaviors you're likely to encounter. Then we'll present what we call the 10 Commandments of Effective Caregiving—a list of basic strategies to help prepare you mentally for the job. Finally, we'll take a nuts-and-bolts look at the day-to-day duties caregiving actually involves, including tips on how these essential tasks can most easily and effectively be performed. It's a lot of work, and important work, so we'd better dig in.

A LITTLE WORSE ALL THE TIME

What might it be like to actually have Alzheimer's disease? Do people with the illness suddenly wake up one day and not know where they are, *who* they are, or who their family members are? Or is the illness more insidious than that, taking the people it affects on a slow but steady journey to oblivion without allowing them as much as a clue?

We wish we could say there's an easy answer to that question, but there's not. "How people with AD perceive their symptoms can be highly individual," says Daniel Kuhn, M.S.W., the education director at the Mather Institute on Aging, who's been working with people with AD for over 25 years.[1] While some people can be agonizingly aware of the changes they experience, others can be nearly blind to them. This degree of awareness can fluctuate dramatically within the same person, moreover, increasing and decreasing from moment to moment as if controlled by some mysterious "dimmer switch," Kuhn says. And just as the inward experiences of AD can be so changeable, so, too, can the outward signs of the illness. A person with Alzheimer's may appear surprisingly normal one moment, only to act lost, confused, agitated, frightened, or even hostile the next.

There simply is no such thing as a typical or consistent pattern for this disease because it can develop so differently in every person it strikes. As explained by John Medina, Ph.D., a professor of molecular biology at the University of Washington School of Medicine and the author of *What You Need to Know About Alzheimer's Disease*, "The most complex organ in the world is undergoing a selective deterioration whose damage cannot be predicted even with the latest medical technology. There will thus be times when the only thing understandable about an AD person's behavior is that it will not be understandable."[2]

For caregivers, of course, this fact can make for one of the greatest challenges you face. Just when you think you've got a particular behavior figured out—another even more bizarre one can come along to take its place. As difficult as this point may be to understand on a personal level, on a biological level it makes perfect sense because Alzheimer's is what's known as a *progressive* disease, meaning it gets a little worse with every passing day, destroying a few more brain cells, deleting a few more "megabytes" of neurological memory. It's true that some people with Alzheimer's disease can appear to remain relatively stable for months, and perhaps even years, but this may not be a true reflection of what's going on inside the brain as AD's infamous plaques and tangles continue to form.

> *While some people can be agonizingly aware of the changes they experience, others can be nearly blind to them. This degree of awareness can fluctuate dramatically within the same person, moreover, increasing and decreasing from moment to moment as if controlled by some mysterious "dimmer switch."*

A BLUNTING OF THE MAGNITUDE— BOTH A BLESSING AND A CURSE

To what degree are people with AD aware of these day-to-day deteriorations happening inside their brains? Again, that depends on the person. Some people can be very aware of the changes and be very upset about them. They know something is beginning to go wrong, but they don't know what. Many people fear they're having a nervous breakdown or going insane and actually are relieved when they learn that what they're experiencing has a physical cause. For others with AD, however, the onset of their illness is more a case of winding up somewhere without quite knowing how they got there. As Kuhn explains, Alzheimer's disease for some people "creates a kind of cushion that softens its meaning for the affected person. It seems that the ability to understand the magnitude of the situation may be blunted by the disease itself."[3]

This isn't to say these people are oblivious to their malady but rather that they become habituated to it—which can be both a blessing and a curse, Kuhn says. A lack of awareness may help protect people with Alzheimer's from the seriousness of what they face, but it also can cause them to be less likely to acknowledge they need help, thus increasing the burdens of those responsible for their care. It can be hard enough to tell Dad he shouldn't drive even when he agrees, for example, but it can be even tougher when he resists tooth and nail.

> *A lack of awareness may help protect people with Alzheimer's from the seriousness of what they face, but it also can cause them to be less likely to acknowledge they need help, thus increasing the burdens of those responsible for their care.*

This is all part of the caregiver's responsibility and the caregiver's challenge, however—to be the voice of reason that our loved ones lose, to be the guardians they may claim not to need. The more that Mom may contend she can still walk alone in the park, the more we may need to hold her hand. The more that Grandpa may still want to cut the grass, the more locks we may need to put on the garage door. Without being disrespectful or patronizing, these are the times that we as caregivers will need to put aside whatever pride our loved ones may want to maintain and get on with our higher duty of keeping them safe.

DON'T NEGATE—ACCOMMODATE

As much as we need to be our loved ones' guardians and protect them from what they can't do, we also need to respect and encourage what they *can* do—which adds yet another level of difficulty to the caregiver's challenge. Good caregiving needs to be "a balancing act," Kuhn says, whereby the person's capabilities are recognized at the same time as their impairments. "Trying to force people with AD into our idea of reality does them a disservice and lowers their self-esteem by emphasizing their limitations instead of their remaining strengths," he adds.[4]

It's better that we "play along" with their idea of the world as much as possible, in other words, and for reasons that can make life easier for us, too. The more we can avoid confrontation and conflict with people with AD, the less agitated, frustrated, and deficient they're apt to feel, and the better their behavior is apt to be. Unlike the way we're accustomed to raising children, "giving in" to people with AD and letting them have their way usually does more good than harm. By helping preserve an environment they understand and in which they feel comfortable and secure, we allow them a peace of mind they may not be able to achieve in any other way.

If Uncle Walt is happy believing he's still in the navy, for example, let him. What's to be gained by denying him that pleasure? Nothing, except agitation for him and perhaps his consequent behavior problems for you. Besides, the fantasy world the person with AD creates may be the only chance for a sense of pride and self-respect, Kuhn points out. By imposing our own versions of reality on the person with AD, we risk denying that person the only chance for dignity and self-respect he or she may have left.

> *The more we can avoid confrontation and conflict with people with AD, the less agitated, frustrated, and deficient they're apt to feel, and the better their behavior is apt to be.*

We could be denying them even more than that, Kuhn adds. Some research suggests that by being tolerant of the fantasy worlds our loved ones may prefer to live in, we allow them a kind of mental enthusiasm that might actually help them resist the effects of their disease. The alternative, which is to shut down their fantasy world, risks doing just the reverse: It may squelch whatever mental excitement they may still be able to muster, perhaps hastening their cognitive decline and making depression more likely as well. Thus, "Don't negate—accommodate" should be our rallying cry as caregivers, even if it does require certain breaches of reality.

THE FUTILITY OF DISCIPLINE: FORGET THE "RIGHTS" AND "WRONGS"

Caregiving, in short, is far more than just baby-sitting. It's baby-sitting made into rocket science because the "rules" often have to be made up as we go. Thankfully, some general principles can guide us in creating these rules, as we'll be seeing shortly, but even these need to be flexible because the behavior of the person with AD can be different from day to day and even hour to hour.

Another difficulty in managing people with this disease is that they usually can't be disciplined in the usual "do this, don't do that" manner we're accustomed to using with children—and for a reason that's frustratingly simple. The reprimand a person with AD receives one minute may not be remembered the next. Discipline by its very nature relies on an ability to remember that most people with AD simply don't have.

Trying to discipline someone with AD, therefore, can be like trying to drive a stake into a pool of water: it's just not going to stick. In fact, attempts at discipline often can backfire, causing the person with AD to act out or become depressed in response to feeling frustration, inadequacy, confusion, or guilt.

The light touch we need to take with our loved ones regarding discipline points to another change in the rules we may need to accept—namely, that the lines between "right" and "wrong" may need to disappear. It may be wrong for 3-year-old Michael to throw his food on the floor, for example, because we can assume he remembers that he's been told not to. With Aunt Meg who's had AD for 5 years, however, we can't make that assumption. We can only assume that something has upset her and then try to figure out what that something is. "You're forever being a detective with this disease," says Martha, who's been taking care of her husband, Ted, for close to 10 years now. "I'm always looking for clues to figuring out what's bothering Ted because it's been quite a while now since he's been able to help me."

THE 10 COMMANDMENTS OF EFFECTIVE CAREGIVING

None of the prior discussion is meant to suggest that people with Alzheimer's disease can't be encouraged to act acceptably, however, because they can, as these basic guidelines will show. We need to remember as we deal with our loved ones with AD, however, that as childlike as they can seem, they shouldn't be treated like children. The goal in managing children and the goal in managing people with AD, after all, are very different. With children, we hope to prepare them for adulthood by teaching them important lessons of life. With people who have Alzheimer's,

> *With people who have Alzheimer's, we're simply trying to make the life they have left as rewarding and meaningful as possible.*

we're simply trying to make the life they have left as rewarding and meaningful as possible. Please consider the following guidelines with that point in mind.

1. Be ready to improvise. There is no such thing as a "typical" case of Alzheimer's disease because there is no such thing as a "typical" human brain. The illness will affect every person differently, and even the same person can be affected differently on different days. The effects of the disease can change even from hour to hour, and there also will be gradual changes as the AD becomes more pronounced over time. Do not, in other words, expect to be able to come up with a single game plan capable of handling any given situation for very long. The person with AD is like a moving target, ever changing, so you'll need to improvise as you go, finding new solutions to new problems at the very moment they arise.

2. Expect the unexpected. As AD progresses, it does increasingly more damage to parts of the brain responsible for personality and the control of inhibitions. As a result, people with this illness may behave in ways that are out of sync, not only for them, but with what society considers acceptable. Such behaviors may include disrobing in public, using inappropriate sexual gestures, displaying seemingly unwarranted emotional outbursts, and making scathing remarks to loved ones or even strangers. Caregivers need to see these behaviors purely as symptoms of the disease, the result of certain neurological connections "shorting out" in the brain.

3. Be sensitive to sensibility. Although these "short-outs" may impair a person's ability to realize the sensibilities of others, people with AD can be left with their own sensibilities well intact. This possibility can be easy for caregivers and family members to overlook, especially if the person with AD appears particularly out of touch. However, often the person with AD can be very "in touch," indeed, and hence may become depressed or angered by demeaning or patronizing remarks he or she may overhear. People with AD often can pick up even on nonverbal cues such body language and the tone of a person's voice, so you and your family may need to be more careful than you realize when conversing in your loved one's presence.

4. Assure security. A defining feature of Alzheimer's disease is its ability to take what was once familiar to a person and make it threateningly strange. Small wonder, then, that people with the illness benefit from constant reassurance that they're safe and well loved. This can be done by reaching out emotionally, with lots of hugs, soothing rubs, and verbal confirmations of love, but also by insuring they feel safe in their physical surroundings and have activities they enjoy doing during the day. Also do your best to keep your loved one's life as simple as possible, because in complexity lies confusion, and in confusion lies the person's anxiety and despair. "It can help to think of the person with AD as a parentless child, because I'm sure that's how they often feel," says Colleen Brooks, R.N., who has made a living of caring for people with AD and other dementias as the owner and chief operator of William's Manor in Wind Gap, Pennsylvania.

5. Strive for peace. As mentioned at the beginning of this chapter, attempts to discipline people with AD usually will do more harm than good by causing them to become even more frustrated, agitated, guilt-ridden, and confused. Your motto, consequently, should be "Make peace, not war" whenever possible. Try to redirect a behavior that is problematic rather than reprimand it, or try to get to the bottom of what's causing the behavior in the first place. This task can be difficult, especially as the disease progresses, but by learning the best ways to communicate with your loved one (as discussed

> *Do your best to keep your loved one's life as simple as possible, because in complexity lies confusion.*

later), you improve your chances of reducing difficult behaviors by eliminating their source. Don't limit your quests for peace just to disciplinary matters, however; also try to avoid playing loud music around your loved one, bustling around to run errands, and having family quarrels. People with AD are easily overstimulated, and problematic behavior often is the result.

6. Sympathize—don't patronize. This tip can be a hard one for some caregivers, especially as AD advances and their loved one may appear in a progressively more regrettable state. Often people with AD will react badly to being talked down to, however, as they still will maintain a sense of dignity, regardless of how helpless they may be. In communicating with your loved one, therefore, speak as you would to any fully functional adult. It can help to keep your sentences relatively short, however, and to use facial gestures and hand motions to emphasize your points. Also try to be sensitive to the degree to which you're being understood. If it appears you may need to repeat something, do so. Remember to be equally helpful as a listener, too. Use facial expressions to show you understand, and don't be afraid to supply a word or concept your loved one may be having trouble with. If you do it in a nonjudgmental manner, he or she will be thankful more than hurt.

> *Often people with AD will react badly to being talked down to—they still will maintain a sense of dignity, regardless of how helpless they may be.*

7. Pacify using the past. Even though recent memories are easily lost by people with AD, often they have an amazing ability to reconnect with their pasts, and they usually will derive a sense of both pleasure and security in doing so. It can be helpful to tap into these archives of good times regularly, especially during periods of inexplicable agitation when there seems to be no discernible cause. Try bringing out old photo albums or records, or simply begin to reminisce about your loved one's fondest times. By going back to the world they can recall, people with AD often will experience, at least temporarily, a resurgence of confidence in dealing with their present one.

8. Let less be more. The urge to want to help our loved ones as much as possible is a natural one—and well intended, of course—but some research suggests we might do better to loosen our grip sometimes and let our loved ones fend more for themselves. This point was shown in a recent study by researchers from the University of Pittsburgh, who found that a group of people with AD in a nursing home learned to dress themselves better—and with less fuss—when their nurses took a more hands-off approach. This example doesn't mean setting up our loved ones for frustration and failure by allowing them to wrestle with tasks beyond their abilities; it does mean having the tolerance and patience to let them try things on their own.[5]

9. Make caregiving a family affair. For the sake of efficiency, it's usually best if one person assumes the role of primary caregiver whose job it is to make most of the day-to-day decisions as well as do most of the day-to-day work of caring for someone with AD. This approach, however, should not exclude enlisting help from other family members or friends whenever possible. If this primary caregiver is you, make a list of all the people who could be available to you, note the ways in which they might be able to help, and keep in regular contact with them about doing just that. Be careful of the trap called "It's probably easiest if I do it myself." That kind of thinking could cause you a breakdown.

> *If you begin to feel overwhelmed emotionally or physically, get help to avoid breaking down entirely.*

10. Know when to ask for help. This may be the most important commandment of all, because your well-being is involved as well as your loved one's. If you begin to feel overwhelmed—emotionally or physically—get help to avoid breaking down entirely. You can start by calling your local chapter of the Alzheimer's Association ([800] 272-3900) and simply explaining your situation. As you'll learn, many services are available to lend you a hand, as the following list shows; some of these are provided by volunteers or government agencies and hence may require no fees. (For more information on these services, see chapter 6.)

- Respite care
- In-home services
- Adult day services
- Retirement housing
- Assisted living facilities
- Skilled nursing facilities
- Continuum care retirement communities
- Hospice care

THE KEY COMPONENTS OF CAREGIVING

We have just taken a look at the basic principles of caregiving for someone with AD. Principles, however, aren't going to get the job done. Action based on knowledge is going to be needed, so get ready to learn what that's going to require. As John Medina, Ph.D., of the University of Washington School of Medicine writes, "This is an illness that can turn the world of the patient upside down." Our goal as caregivers should be to try as much as we can to turn it right side up.[6]

Hygiene and Personal Care

These aspects of caregiving can be the most difficult of all, for caregivers and care getters alike—difficult for caregivers because these are not tasks we're used to performing for another adult, and difficult for our loved ones with AD because it constitutes an invasion of their privacy as well as proof of just how dependent on another person they've become. These aspects of caregiving are important for cosmetic reasons as well as good health, however, so they mustn't be slighted, unpleasant as they may be. Here are some helpful tips from the Alzheimer's Association for making these daily duties go as smoothly as possible.

Bathing

Regular bathing is important, not only to keep your loved one looking and smelling his or her best but also to minimize risks of skin infection and infection in the genital area. You should pay special attention to this latter area, in fact, and alert your loved one's doctor if you notice any rashes or sores beginning to form. Know, too, that if there's a time your loved one may be prone to acting out, this is it. For reasons not fully understood, bathing seems to be particularly stressful for people with AD, but you can minimize their discomfort in these ways:

> *Bathing seems to be particularly stressful for people with AD, but you can minimize their discomfort.*

- Allow your loved one to decide the time of day he or she prefers to be bathed and whether by shower or tub.

- Have everything ready in advance—proper room temperature, water temperature, soaps, and towels.

- Be sure adequate rubber mats are in place to prevent slips, and have handrails installed along the sides of the tub or shower if they seem required.

- Allow your loved one to hide behind a towel as much as possible if he or she seems embarrassed to be seen nude.

- When washing your loved one's hair, use a washcloth to do the soaping and rinsing to avoid excess water contacting the face. People with AD tend to be hypersensitive to water and, much like small children, in the area of the face, especially.

- Be gentle when toweling, using pats rather than rubs to get your loved one dry.

- Don't feel a bath is needed every day, especially if it constitutes a struggle. Two or three days a week may be enough if sponge baths are given in between.

Teeth Brushing

If your loved one is capable of handling this task, count yourself lucky and hope this ability lasts. Many people with AD will lose this seemingly elementary capability, however, because it involves several steps. Here's how to help if you notice your loved one neglecting this important chore or doing an inadequate job:

- As with bathing, try to establish a routine that accommodates your loved one's least resistant moods. It may be better to brush when you can, in other words, rather than to struggle with the task after every meal.

- Give basic instructions, and then let your loved one do as much as possible by him- or herself.

- If your loved one wears dentures, remove these at night and give them a good cleaning, being sure to check with your loved one's dentist if you're not sure how. Brush your loved one's gums and the roof of the mouth at this time, too, keeping an eye open for any sores on the gums and alerting your loved one's dentist if any are present.

- If your loved one defiantly refuses to open up, try at least to brush the fronts of the teeth, and talk to your loved one's dentist about the problem. Products are available such as props to hold the mouth open as well as dental foams, peroxide solutions, and mouthwashes that can do a reasonable job in the place of a conventional brushing.

Grooming

Like so many other aspects of caregiving, grooming the person with AD requires compromise. You want your loved one to look well enough to feel good, but you don't want to drive yourself crazy trying to achieve a well-kept appearance. Here are some suggestions with that goal in mind:

- Go short. Suggest a hairstyle that is as short and easy to manage as possible. If your loved one is female and has been used to and still enjoys visiting a hairdresser for the maintenance of a more elaborate hairdo, however, do your best to accommodate that routine.

- Use the sink rather than tub for washing hair. This approach can be easier on your back because you won't need to bend as much, and you can make the job even easier with a hose that attaches to the faucet.

- Go electric when shaving. Whether you're doing a man's face or a woman's legs, an electric razor is much safer than a manual.

- Don't forget the nails. Neglected finger- and toenails can become ingrown before the person with AD might have the wherewithal to notice.

- Discourage makeup. It can be exasperating to apply, but if your loved one insists and it helps her feel better about herself, do what you can. Often just some facial powder and lipstick can be enough.

Dressing

As much as we take this basic activity for granted, it can involve sequences of tasks that the person with AD can find overwhelming, especially as the illness becomes more severe. As with the other aspects of personal maintenance, let your loved one do as much possible, and offer help only if you notice the person becoming too frustrated to finish the job. These suggestions should help:

- Lay the clothes to be worn out on your loved one's bed, placing the garments from left to right in the order they're to be put on. If your loved one is the type to be fussy, you might want to offer two options for each exterior garment. More than that could only make the person with AD more confused.

- Eliminate unneeded accessories such as scarfs, vests, belts, and jewelry. They will add to your loved one's confusion and hence indecision and only require more time and frustration to be donned. Also, reduce the size of your loved one's wardrobe in general: a closet filled with decades of options is an invitation to confusion.

- Find what's easiest to work with. If your loved one resists having clothing pulled down over the face, opt for garments that button or zipper. Velcro fasteners tend to be the easiest to manage of all.

- Avoid shoes that are difficult to buckle or tie. Shoes that slip on or fasten with Velcro are best. Make sure they're a good fit and don't have slippery soles that pose a risk for falls.

- Go for the baggy look. Not only is it hip, it's easiest to get on and off.

- Don't be a fashion critic. If the ensembles your loved one feels most comfortable in are a bit of a stretch in terms of good taste, relax. You can help guard against such truly horrific combinations, however, by buying clothes that are difficult to mismatch in the first place—lots of solid colors that work well in a variety of combinations instead of potentially disastrous patterns and plaids.

- Tolerate monotony. If your loved one likes wearing the same outfit every day, buy it in duplicate or triplicate if need be. Better that the person is happy than impeccably dressed.

Mealtime

Meals can offer the greatest challenge of all to caregivers, for several reasons. Not only may people with AD forget how to sit at the table and use basic tableware, but they may forget even what to do with a bite of food once it's in their mouth. They also can be very finicky about what they eat and be prone to throwing their food, sometimes on the floor, sometimes at other people. At the other extreme, however, people with this disease may forget when they've eaten and want to eat almost constantly. Hiding food in odd places around the house can be another problem, as can perhaps the most alarming behavior of all—eating nonnutritive items around the house such as paper, house plants, or soap, as the person may lose the ability to distinguish between what's edible and what's not.

> *Meals can offer the greatest challenge of all to caregivers. Not only may people with AD forget how to sit at the table and use basic tableware, but they may forget even what to do with a bite of food once it's in their mouth.*

Not all people with AD will have such difficulties eating, so don't panic at these possibilities. Do be prepared for them, however, and consider these basic strategies for keeping mealtime as "normal" as possible:

- Strive for a regular eating schedule, with a minimum of activity or confusion that the person with AD could find distracting.

- Use solid-colored plates (patterns can be confusing) that provide a contrast with the place mat or table so as to be more easily seen. Also remove any objects from the table that your loved one might find distracting such as candles, a centerpiece, salt and pepper shakers, or a sugar bowl.

- Do your best to serve foods that your loved one likes but that also will provide good nutrition. Also be sure that the foods being served have had ample time to cool.

- If your loved one wears dentures, make sure they're comfortable and snug.

- Reduce confusion by serving just one food at a time—the meat separately from the vegetables or potatoes, for example—and be sure to cut foods that need to be chewed into small pieces to reduce the risk of choking.

> *Reduce confusion by serving just one food at a time—the meat separately from the vegetables or potatoes, for example.*

- Do not scold if your loved one finds it easier to eat with his or her hands. Good nutrition needs to take precedence over table manners.

- Consider fitting your loved one with a bib or smock to protect clothing.

- Purchase special nonslip plates at a medical supply store if the ones you're using won't stay put, or try putting a damp cloth beneath plates to keep them from sliding.

- If drinking from a glass becomes troublesome, purchase special no-spill cups available for small children.

- If your loved one begins hoarding food, try making nutritious foods available throughout the day.

- Be sure your loved one is getting enough fluids (ask your loved one's doctor how much this should be), and limit caffeinated beverages such as coffee, tea, and colas to about 8 ounces a day. (Caffeine is a diuretic that can encourage frequent urination.)

- If your loved one is taking a medication that has dry mouth as a side effect, remember to offer liquids frequently as the person eats to make swallowing easier.

- If chewing is a problem for your loved one, puree meals in a blender or food processor, and feed with a spoon. Also be careful not to let your loved one have foods such as hard candies, nuts, carrots, chewing gum, or popcorn that could cause choking. (If choking does occur, stand behind your loved one, grab around the waist, locking your hands just below the ribs, and give a good yank. Repeat this technique as often as necessary until whatever is caught has been dislodged.)

- Keep track of your loved one's weight, and notify his or her doctor should any significant gains or losses occur.

- Pay attention to good nutrition, which is just as important for people with AD as it is for anyone else. Nutritional shortages can increase risks of many physical illnesses and infections and could even exacerbate the confusion so characteristic of AD. According to the American Dietetic Association, people of all ages should eat foods from each of the five major food groups every day. As the Food Guide Pyramid in figure 4.1 shows, this advice means two to three servings of a high-calcium dairy products such as milk, cheese, yogurt, or cottage cheese; two to three servings of a high-protein food such as beef, pork, fish, poultry, eggs, dried beans, or nuts; three to five servings of vegetables; two to four servings of fruit; and eight to 11 servings of whole-grain cereals, pasta, or bread. The number of servings will depend on the person's size and how physically active he or she is. If mealtime remains unmanageable despite your most ardent efforts, check with your local chapter of the Alzheimer's Association to see what programs might be available in your area to help out.

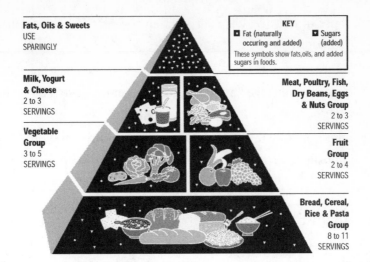

Figure 4.1—*The Food Guide Pyramid*

Source: Centers for Disease Control and Prevention

Toilet Duties

Certainly not the most pleasant caregiving responsibility, overseeing your loved one's processes of elimination is vital, nonetheless. Regular elimination of waste is important for good health, but it can present problems for people with AD as their illness becomes more advanced. These folks may move too slowly to get to the bathroom in time, they may be unable to unbutton or unzip themselves in the ways required, or they may simply have trouble remembering from day to day how to get the bathroom at all. It's important for caregivers to be attentive to these potential obstacles and provide the appropriate assistance so that accidents don't occur. Slip-ups not only can be unpleasant for caregivers to deal with but also can be hard on the self-esteem of their perpetrators, too. Here's how to keep toilet-related traumas to a minimum:

- Keep a record of the times of day your loved one needs to urinate or have a bowel movement, and look for a pattern. If one exists, make efforts to escort your loved one to the bathroom at those times to lessen the risk of an accident (see the sidebar "Inroads Against Incontinence").

- As with a small child, watch for visual cues such as facial expressions or fidgeting that could indicate your loved one needs "to go."

- Mark the way to the bathroom, perhaps with brightly colored (nonslip) throw rugs, and remove anything such as a waste-

Inroads Against Incontinence

Incontinence. The word itself strikes fear in caregivers, and understandably so. It's a natural human reaction to be repulsed by excrement, especially when it's not our own. The involuntary production of human waste in both its forms is often an unavoidable feature of Alzheimer's disease, however, and needs to be dealt with. Fortunately, the causes of both urinary and fecal incontinence sometimes are medical ones that can be treated, so don't assume the worst until you've had your loved one examined should accidents begin to occur.

Know, too, that urinary and fecal incontinence are entirely separate medical conditions, due to unrelated causes. While urinary incontinence may be due to a bladder infection, diabetes, the side effect of a medication, enlargement of the prostate in men, or—surprisingly—dehydration, the possible causes of fecal incontinence are different: an infection of the bowels, diarrhea, constipation, or a potentially more serious condition called *impaction* in which the large intestine becomes blocked completely. (These last two conditions might seem like the last things to cause incontinence, but their danger is that they can interfere with a person's ability to control the urge to have a bowel movement if and when it finally does arrive.)

So what can be done to stem the tide against incontinence? Tips included in the basic tutorial on toileting given earlier should help, but here are some additional ideas should those fall short:

paper basket from nearby the toilet to reduce risks of that being used instead.

- Provide sources of entertainment in the bathroom such as books, magazines, or music to encourage your loved one to invest the time elimination may take.

- Consider having support devices professionally installed on either side of the toilet so that your loved one not only can

---

- For urinary incontinence, check with your loved one's doctor to determine the amount of fluid that should be consumed daily.

- If bed-wetting is a problem, limit fluid intake in the evening hours.

- Use night-lights to make the path to the bathroom clear.

- Initiate regular visits to the bathroom every several hours even if your loved one doesn't have to go.

- If initiating urination is a problem for your loved one, have him or her blow bubbles in a glass of water with a straw. This method often can help.

- To guard couches and chairs, have them fitted with washable slipcovers, and protect their cushions by inserting them into an appropriately sized plastic trash bag.

Remember, though, that incontinence is one of the major reasons caregivers decide they no longer can care for their loved ones at home, so don't feel bad if it becomes an insurmountable problem despite your having tried these tips. As Alzheimer's Association consultant and expert in caregiver stress Avrene Brandt, Ph.D., says, "There is a limit to how much one person can reasonably be asked to do for another, and caregivers need to know when their limit has been reached."

support him- or herself should things take a while but also has an easier time of getting on and off the toilet without the indignity of needing help.

The Pros and Cons of Diapers

Should you protect against accidents by encouraging your loved one to wear what amounts to an adult diaper—also called adult briefs— sold in pharmacies and medical supply stores? The verdict is split on this issue. While some experts feel these disposable garments can significantly reduce worry for caregivers and their loved ones alike, others argue they demean the person with AD in addition to risking resistance that can make them more trouble than they're worth. What

---

Solving the "Sundowning" Syndrome

For reasons not fully understood, people with AD and other dementias tend to be the most difficult to manage in the late afternoon and early evening—usually between the hours of approximately 3 P.M. and 7 P.M.—hence the term *sundowning*. Perhaps it's because they get cranky from fatigue, or they feel less secure when daylight fades, or they become jealous if their primary caregiver begins showing attention to other family members arriving home from school or work. Sometimes the excitement of extra family activity at night can upset people with AD, too. Whatever the reason, don't be surprised if your loved one tends to be more agitated, more needy, and more apt to act out during this time—bad timing, indeed, considering this is when you're apt to be edgy from fatigue, too.

Fortunately, there are ways sundowning can be minimized, so if it becomes a problem, give one or more of the following suggestions a try:

- Make sure your loved one is getting enough exercise during the day to help get tuckered out naturally.

experts do agree on, however, is that only the caregiver can make the final call. If diapers would seem to make your life easier and your loved one isn't opposed, they can be well worth the expense. If their application would be even more trouble than what they're designed to prevent, however, don't feel you're missing out on any particularly state-of-the-art form of control. If you're uncertain about this matter, get the opinion of your loved one's doctor.

KEEPING YOUR LOVED ONE SAFE

Safety can be a major concern, and rightfully so. People with this illness often will maintain physical capabilities far beyond their mental

- Try to get your loved one to take a short nap after lunch so he or she won't be so tired later, or encourage the person to stay in bed longer in the morning.

- Offer a healthful afternoon snack such as fruit or yogurt to prevent late-afternoon energy slumps.

- Try to soothe your loved one's agitation with music he or she might especially enjoy or the scent of lavender oil, which can help calm people with AD, says Frena Gray-Davidson, the director of Self-Help Alzheimer's Caregiver's Training and Information (SHACTI).[7]

- If possible, separate family activity from where your loved one spends time in the evening to prevent overstimulation.

- If a want of attention could be your loved one's problem as you tend to family affairs, try to find activities that might be of interest, such as looking at photo albums, listening to old records, watching a favorite TV show, or doing a soothingly repetitive task such as sorting socks or folding laundry.

ones, which can be a recipe for disaster. One caregiver tells of how her 80-year-old mother managed to scale an 8-foot-high wrought iron fence in subfreezing temperatures and wound up an hour's drive from home, wearing nothing but a nightgown. At the other extreme, some people with AD can become feeble to the point of being at serious risk for falls. Then, too, poor judgment is a defining feature of this disease, which renders most household appliances accidents waiting to happen. Every person with AD is different, of course, and the stage of your loved one's illness also is an important factor, but here are precautions that are generally wise to take.

At Home

This is where most accidents happen, especially in the kitchen and bathroom. Here's how to keep your home the sanctuary it needs to be.

In the kitchen. Sharp objects and the stove are the greatest dangers here, but appliances such as toaster ovens, portable electric grills, hot plates, blenders, and electric mixers can pose hazards, too. Keep all potentially dangerous utensils and appliances out of reach or under lock and key, and remove knobs from your stove or cover them with childproof guards.

In the bathroom. More falls occur in the bathroom than any other room of the house, so make sure all rugs and mats have slip-resistant backings, and consider having handrails installed if you think they would make it easier for your loved one to use the bathtub, shower, or toilet. Also be sure to keep all potentially dangerous medications well out of reach, and reduce the temperature of your hot water so that it's not hot enough to scald.

Up and down the stairs. Make sure stairways are well lit and that handrails and any carpeting or stair pads are firmly attached. If your loved one is incapable of safely using the stairs at all, install the type of gates used to protect small children at the head of stairways.

On the floor. Keep floors free of clutter and extension cords, make sure rugs don't slip, and go easy on the high-gloss waxes on tiled or linoleum surfaces.

In the cabinets. Keep all potentially hazardous products such as pesticides, paints, cleaners, and solvents in cabinets that are either locked or held closed by childproof latches. Ditto for guns and potentially hurtful items such as saws, hammers, and nails.

Doors and windows. In some cases, it may be advisable to install locks on all doors and windows to keep someone with AD safely put. (Be sure you and other family members know where these keys are kept, however, in the event that an emergency evacuation might be needed, such as in the case of a fire.) For some rooms such as bathrooms and bedrooms, on the other hand, it may be a good idea to remove locks to prevent the person with AD from locking themselves *in*.

Outdoors. It's important to keep porches, patios, decks, and yards safe, too. Protect glass storm doors with visible grillwork. Make glass patio doors more discernible with some sort of visible decals. Ensure that all railings around elevated porches and decks are in good shape. Install banisters along outside steps, and paint them in bright colors. Never leave someone with AD in the vicinity of an outdoor grill that's in use, lock away all potentially dangerous garden tools, and if you have a swimming pool, be extra careful *never* to leave a person with AD alone in its vicinity.

> *Fortunately, many people with AD lose their desire to smoke as their disease progresses; in fact, they may simply forget they ever had the habit at all.*

If your loved one smokes. Here's a loaded gun for sure—a fire risk and health risk all in one. Fortunately, many people with AD lose their desire to smoke as their disease progresses; in fact, they may simply forget they ever had the habit at all. If not, do everything you can to get your loved one to quit or at least demand that you always be present if and when they do smoke.

If your loved one drinks alcohol. This, too, can be a hazardous combination given alcohol's propensity for impairing judgment—a problem for the person with AD, of course, even before they take their first sip. As with smoking, try to get your loved one to quit or at least to cut down. If this doesn't work, try at least to be present when they imbibe.

Don't let yourself be a hazard. "It has been shown that accidents are much more likely to occur in the home if the caregiver is angry or in a hurry," says Medina, the author of *What You Need to Know About Alzheimer's Disease*. His advice? "Slow down; take time to change the atmosphere to a more relaxed state."[8]

Don't forget the ID. This is one of the simplest but most important precautionary measures caregivers can take. Talk to your loved one's doctor about having an identification bracelet or necklace made up that gives your loved one's name, address, and phone number, and mentions that they suffer from Alzheimer's disease, a memory disorder that could prevent the person from knowing where he or she lives if found away from home. This precaution can greatly facilitate your loved one's safe and speedy return home.

On the Road

At what point should someone with AD be prevented from driving? In light of research showing that 40 percent of people diagnosed with the illness are involved in an auto accident in the 6 months prior to being diagnosed, the answer would seem to be "the sooner the better."[9] These results shouldn't be surprising given the complex motor skill and good judgment safe driving requires. Current laws are lagging far behind the danger AD poses on our highways, however, so you may need to be aggressive to have your loved one's driving privileges revoked should you feel it necessary.

Start by calling the Department of Motor Vehicles to find out what's required in your state. If you're lucky, a written statement from your loved one's doctor stating the patient's incompetence will be enough. In some states, however, the process is far more complicated and may even be legally impossible. If this is the case and you're convinced your loved one is a hazard to him- or herself and others, it may be necessary for you simply to take safety into your own hands and "pull the keys," meaning you'll physically need take away your loved one's car keys. If for some reason that approach is not possible, you may have to resort to rendering your loved one's car inoperable, something you can do easily enough by detaching the car's distributor cap, a small device responsible for the firing of the engine's spark plugs. No damage done and possibly some lives saved. Ask a mechanic to show you how.

Forty percent of people diagnosed with AD are involved in an auto accident in the 6 months prior to being diagnosed.

How do you decide that a person with AD is, in fact, unfit to drive? You can have your loved one undergo a neurological examination for the purpose of that determination, but you also can look for clues, some obvious, some less so. Frequent traffic citations and fender benders are no-brainers that your loved one's driving skills are waning, but also look for more subtle signs such as the following:

- Your loved one easily gets lost when driving.
- Your loved one has been driving noticeably more slowly lately.
- Your loved is quick to get angry and blame other drivers for miscues when, in fact, the fault lies closer to home.
- Your loved one prefers not to have others in the car when driving (to avoid being exposed).
- Your loved one's miscues and inabilities around the house have you concerned he or she could be a danger behind the wheel.

If the writing on the wall does seem to be that your loved one shouldn't be behind the wheel, don't prepare for a struggle until there actually is one. Often people with AD will realize their inadequacy and be frightened by it as much as anyone else. They also may be unaware or in denial about it, however, in which case you'll need to be diplomatic. Start by honestly expressing your concern for your loved one's safety—and the safety of others on the highway. If that route gets you nowhere, go to your loved one's doctor, explain the reasons for your concern, and let the physician try to convince your loved one of the risks being incurred. Explain to your loved one, too, that if driving is continued after being given a medical warning not to, you, the caregiver, could be held legally responsible for any harm that may result.

> *L*oss of driving privileges can constitute a very hurtful blow for people with AD, as a symbol of just how impaired and dependent on others they've become.

Loss of driving privileges can constitute a very hurtful blow for people with AD, as a symbol of just how impaired and dependent on others they've become. But far better that pride be lost than life.

KEEPING YOUR LOVED ONE ENTERTAINED

"A dementing illness does not mean an end to enjoying life," write Nancy L. Mace, M.A., and Peter V. Rabins, M.D., M.P.H., in their aptly named caregiver's guide, *The 36-Hour Day*.[10] What the dementing illness *can* mean, however, is that you as a caregiver will need to take responsibility for your loved one's enjoyment of life because he or she no longer can. You will need to be your loved one's "tour guide" in the years ahead, in a sense, an entertainment director ready and willing to fit enjoyable activities into the day. It might not always be easy, demanding imagination and patience based on a regimen of trial and error, but trust that your efforts can be well worth it—for you and your loved one alike.

No one knows your loved one as well as you do, of course, so these suggestions will need to be fine-tuned. Even if you get discouraged, know that for people with AD, even just a little can mean a lot. Their world has been much reduced, so it can easily be enhanced. Here are some ideas to get you thinking:

- As with exercise, try to find activities you and your loved one can do enjoyably together.

- Plan activities for times of the day when your loved one is well rested, not tired or cranky.

- Keep activities simple and repetitive, but be careful not to demean your loved one by suggesting activities that are overtly childish, such as coloring or playing with dolls. Often the person with AD will have the sense to take offense.

- Find out what card games, board games, or crossword puzzles your loved one still might enjoy. Games that your loved one may have liked during youth might have special staying power.

- Determine the degree to which your loved one still is able to read, and make appropriate reading materials available such as favorite books, newspapers, and magazines.

- Tap into the power of music. It's rare for a person with AD not to appreciate this uniquely emotional art form, especially tunes that can help the person reminisce. See whether your loved one can operate a tape deck, CD player, or radio so he or she can enter the world of music independently.

> *Keep activities simple and repetitive, but be careful not to demean your loved one by suggesting activities that are overtly childish.*

- Take music to a higher level by encouraging your loved one to sing or dance, with you or as a "solo" act—whichever seems most effective.

- If your loved one once played a musical instrument, encourage that activity, too. (Be careful not to be too pushy here, however, as the degree to which a person's skills may have declined could be too upsetting to accept. Have this consideration for other former skills, too, such as artwork, photography, needlework, or writing.)

- Suggest outings such shopping trips, sightseeing, eating out, or simply taking rides in the car to provide variety to your loved one's day—and yours as well. If such outings seem only to confuse, however, you may need to find a sitter for your loved one so that you can enjoy these important diversions alone.

- Allow your loved one the chance to "help" with simple chores around the house such as dusting, drying dishes, folding laundry, digging in the garden, stacking firewood, or raking leaves. Be prepared for a short attention span, and never encourage activities that could do harm.

- Arrange for your loved one to see old friends as much as possible if such visits give joy. Warn these friends ahead of time, however, that short visits may be best, and note that not more than one or two people should visit at a time to reduce overstimulation.

> *Consider allowing the pleasure of a pet. Many cats and dogs, interestingly, will show a special kind of affection for people with AD and other dementias.*

- If your loved one has been fond of animals in the past, consider allowing the pleasure of a pet. Many cats and dogs, interestingly, will show a special kind of affection for people with AD and other dementias.

- Take time simply to sit and let your loved one reminisce about his or her fondest memories, perhaps looking at old photographs or listening to old songs as you do. The past is often where people with AD feel most comfortable, after all, so we should allow them this pleasure as often as we can.

- Provide opportunities for your loved one to enjoy experiences that stimulate the senses—sight, taste, touch, hearing, and smell—in basic ways. Go for walks or car rides at sunrise or sunset; let the person smell fresh flowers, hear birds sing, taste favorite foods, or rub a texture that may be particularly pleasing, such as felt, fur, or even just a smooth piece of wood.

- Perhaps most important of all, try not to forget the universal comfort derived from human contact—rubbing, hugging, or simply holding hands. As words become less effective in the later stages of this disease, these forms of communication can become more so.

- Finally, don't feel you need to go it alone. Consider using family members, friends, or even an adult day care center or in-home visitor program to give yourself what could be a much-needed break. The variety sometimes can be good for the person with AD as well.

KEEPING YOUR LOVED ONE FIT

"It's the best part of our day," says Susan of the time she and her mother spend on their afternoon walks. "Mom looks so forward to getting outside, and it almost always puts her in a better mood. Besides, it's great for putting me in a better mood, too."

Exercise can be amazing medicine, all right, so by all means do the best you can to include at least 20 minutes of some sort of physical activity in your loved one's day. Exercise for people with AD can benefit both their minds and bodies, and it can do the same for caregivers (see chapter 5). Daily exercise for people with Alzheimer's may help them sleep better, feel less restless and agitated, be less apt to wander, feel less depressed, and maybe even think more clearly. Exercise does need to be presented and supervised in the right ways, however, because the person with AD, of course, is not the typical fitness consumer looking for a sexier physique. That said, here are some tips from Jamie Clark, the president of the Senior Fitness Association (SFA), plus other fitness experts on how to work more physical activity into your loved one's day:

> *Exercise for people with AD can benefit both their minds and bodies, and it can do the same for caregivers.*

- Find activities your loved one enjoys. Often people with AD will retain a fondness for activities they pursued with some proficiency in their youth.

- Realize that yard work and household chores can be valuable forms of exercise, so encourage these activities—and also supervise them—whenever possible.

- Accompany your loved one in the activity if possible. Not only can this approach allow the person with AD to mimic your actions should the activity be at all tricky like bowling or tennis, it can be a good chance to bond.

- Schedule the activity at the same time every day to help establish a routine, but be sure it's a time when your loved one is in an appropriate mood.

Age Is No Barrier to Fitness Benefits

"We can't stop Mother Natures' clock, but we can slow it down," says senior fitness expert Mary Ann Wilson, R.N., the originator and host of public television's popular half-hour exercise show for the elderly called *Sit and Be Fit*. And it's not heavy-duty huffing and puffing Wilson is talking about. "General physical activity, not just structured exercise, can help promote many important health benefits," she says.[11]

Better yet, these benefits are just as available for people with AD as they are for the rest of us, says Patrick J. Bird, Ph.D., of the College of Health and Human Performance at the University of Florida. "People with Alzheimer's disease can derive physiological and psychological benefits from exercise that are similar to those gained by healthy individuals," Dr. Bird says. "There is even some evidence that exercise may improve the ability of people with Alzheimer's disease to communicate."[12]

For more on that good news, see chapter 5. In the meantime, check out these exercise benefits—to be enjoyed by both people with AD and their caregivers:

- Never try to force your loved one to exercise. It may be permissible and sometimes even necessary to encourage or entice your loved one, but force usually will just cause a person to resist even more strongly.

- Put a premium on simplicity. This means avoiding activities that could frustrate your loved one and hence squelch interest. Walking often is a great choice for people with AD for this reason.

- Be sensitive to your loved one's fatigue and attention span. It may be best to divide exercise time into two or three sessions

- Improvements in cardiovascular fitness by as much as 25 percent
- Increases in muscle strength (One study done at Tufts University found that elderly people were able to increase their strength by 175 percent in just 8 weeks.)[13]
- Improved flexibility
- Lower risk of heart disease
- Lower risk of diabetes
- Lower blood pressure
- Less constipation
- Less body fat and more lean muscle tissue
- Stronger immunity
- Prevention of bone loss
- Reductions in anxiety, insomnia, and depression

Note: For information on how to obtain a series of exercise videocassettes called *Movement in Nature,* tailored to the needs of people with Alzheimer's disease, contact TBA Communications, 152 Simsbury Road, Box 677, Avon, CT 06001 (Phone: [800] 345-2689).

that will add up to 20 to 30 minutes rather than going for it all at once.

- Take time to warm up. Even if you're just walking, it's important to start out slowly and increase your speed progressively to give muscles a chance to warm up. The same goes with cooling down: Don't stop all at once, but rather slow down gradually.

- Consider taking your loved one along with you to an exercise or yoga class, or exercise together to a fitness program on videotape or TV. (See the discussion on *Sit and Be Fit* and *Movement in Nature* in the sidebar "Age Is No Barrier to Fitness Benefits.")

- Be sure to get medical approval before engaging your loved one in an exercise program. As healthful as exercise generally is, it could be dangerous under certain medical conditions.

IMPROVING COMMUNICATION

"He took his nourishment well, but had great annoyance from his inability to find the words he wished for," wrote the son of American poet Ralph Waldo Emerson—just one of the many great minds to suffer from Alzheimer's disease over the ages. For a poet, of course, it was the cruelest blow.[14]

Alzheimer's disease also can be unkind for caregivers, however, as they attempt to decipher the needs and desires of their lost-for-words loved ones. Not only may people with AD have trouble finding the right word; they may invent words of their own, use words inappropriately, revert to using curse words out of frustration, repeat certain favorite words that make sense only to them, or simply give up and not speak at all.

Communication can present quite a challenge for caregivers. To improve your chances of making sense of what may at times appear to be anything but, follow these tips from the Alzheimer's Association.

When listening. Maintain eye contact, show in your facial expressions that you're sincere in trying to understand, and be careful not to interrupt. If the person appears to be struggling over a particular word or concept, however, politely try to help out. Be calm and supportive in assisting the person, using a relaxed and friendly tone of voice.

When speaking. Always face the person and speak slowly and clearly but not in a tone that seems obviously patronizing. Use hand gestures and facial expressions to help get your points across, use specific names of people rather than pronouns such as he or she, and try to keep your sentences short. Also feel free to hold the person's hand when speaking or listening. It's amazing how communicative we can be through our nonverbal power of touch.

RESPONDING TO CHALLENGING BEHAVIORS

The list can read like a "who's who" in annoyance: clinging, complaining, accusing, wandering, hoarding, rummaging, physical aggression, defiance, sexual improprieties, stubbornness, and, perhaps the most irksome of all, repeating the same question over and over and over again. Making a challenging situation even harder is that such behaviors often will be very much out of character for the way the person acted before developing Alzheimer's.

So how do you as a caregiver keep your cool day after day in the face of such aggravation? Experts from the Alzheimer's Association have given this a lot of thought, fortunately, and have come up with some helpful suggestions. First, continually remind yourself that it's the illness that's making your loved one act this way. Just as a cold can make someone sneeze or cough, Alzheimer's disease can make someone a "pain-in-the-neck," to put it mildly. We can minimize this pain by doing our best to be analytical about the situation, by taking the following steps:

1. Try to determine the cause. Because people with AD often can't effectively verbalize what's bothering them, you may have to be a bit of a detective. Usually the cause of aggravation will fall into one of several categories: your loved one could be feeling physically uncomfortable, overstimulated by a noisy or chaotic environment, ill, threatened by an unfamiliar environment, frustrated by too complicated a task or an inability to communicate, or angry about having been disallowed something or having overheard a disparaging remark.

2. Try to find a solution. Trial and error may need to be your primary method, but be persistent because most problematic behaviors can be solved. Analyze what may have brought the behavior on. Also analyze how you first reacted to the behavior. Sometimes a caregiver's aggravated response to a particular behavior can be as upsetting for the person with AD as whatever may have flustered the person in the first place. Try to be as calm and understanding as possible, and gently ask questions that might help determine the cause of your loved one's unrest. Does he or she want something, or is the person hungry, uncomfortable, confused, or angry?

> *Because people with AD often can't effectively verbalize what's bothering them, you may have to be a bit of a detective.*

3. Temper your temper. Can't you just forcefully tell people with AD that they're misbehaving, you may be wondering, and that they will be punished if they don't stop, much as you would discipline a small child? You can try, but you're unlikely to get anywhere and probably will only make the person more upset. In the words of Jamie Clark, who has worked with many people with AD over the years, "As long as your loved one's safety is not at risk, it does not pay to resist, contradict, correct, criticize, argue, or debate." This approach can seem like the direct opposite of how we're taught to discipline our children, but our goal in managing people with AD, we must remember, is very different. There can be no teaching of appropriate behavior or important life lessons because there can be no teaching at all.

This situation can be very frustrating for caregivers, but it needs to be accepted as the reality of this disease. Lack of responsiveness in people with AD can cause many caregivers to want to "blow their stacks," and while the feeling is a natural one, it's also one that's important to control. It may be permissible to lose your temper occasionally, but if this reaction starts to become frequent—especially if it's accompanied by hitting, shoving, or in some way constraining the person with AD—it's a sign you need help. Call the Alzheimer's Association if this behavior happens, and ask about getting relief through an adult day care center or part-time sitter. Not everyone is cut out to be a full-time caregiver, remember, and the chore can be especially difficult if the person you're caring for is someone you have never particularly liked. Don't risk your mental well-being—or the physical well-being of the person with AD—if you find the task is simply too much. Get help or find someone else to handle the job.

> *Lack of responsiveness in people with AD can cause many caregivers to want to "blow their stacks," and while the feeling is a natural one, it's also one that's important to control.*

The Top 10 Most Difficult Behaviors and What to Do About Them

Every person with AD will act differently, of course, but here are behaviors caregivers generally find the most difficult to manage, plus some ideas for addressing them:

1. Nighttime wandering. Though wandering can occur during the day as a result of general disorientation with the person's surroundings, wandering at night tends to be both more troublesome and more dangerous. To control it, make sure the person with AD is getting enough exercise during the day so he or she will be apt to sleep better at night. Also restrict napping in the afternoon, which could be causing restlessness at night, and talk to your loved one's doctor about the appropriate use of medications to limit late-night meanderings. Be sure to keep windows and doors locked, and install gates at the top

The Caregiver's Challenge:
To Give Even When the Giving Gets Tough

In the same way that comedian Rodney Dangerfield complains he "can't get any respect," as a caregiver for someone with AD, you may find thanks to be in short supply. This won't mean the appreciation isn't there but rather that it could be buried beneath too much confusion and fear to come out.

Many caregivers find this situation difficult to accept, and understandably so. Caregiving requires tremendous amounts of time and devotion, yet the only thanks you get could be a temper tantrum, a kick in the shins, or a bowl of soup in the face. These behaviors have distinct neurological causes, as we'll be examining more closely later in this chapter, but they can still hurt, physically as well as emotionally. These are the times you'll need to reach back for that something extra, as the saying goes, and accept that dealing with such behaviors is all part of the caregiver's challenge of learning to give even when the giving gets tough.

of stairs to prevent falls. As a last resort, you may need to consider the use of a special chair or bed designed to help keep your wayward loved one put.

2. **Hoarding and hiding.** Why these behaviors are common for people with AD is not clear, but they sure can be inconvenient, such as when you can't find the car keys or your loved one's dentures. People with AD may hoard food, which can become a sanitation problem. There's not a lot that can be done about hoarding, unfortunately, other than learning to outsmart it or live with it. If your loved one insists on putting the silverware under a couch cushion, for example, that may have to be the new place for the silverware. And if your

loved one needs to keep a stash of food in a dresser drawer, allow some in that spot, and be sure to renew the supply so it stays fresh. Otherwise, make special efforts to keep valuable or potentially dangerous items such as money, jewelry, sharp knives, and firearms under lock and key or well out of reach. You also might want to get into the habit of checking wastepaper baskets before emptying them.

3. Clinging and following. Some people with AD will want to cling to their caregivers like a shadow, following them even into the bathroom. The reason, basically, is that the caregiver may represent the only source of security the person with AD has. Another factor is that the person with AD may simply not be able to remember that the caregiver will be coming back, so the safest thing is just not to let the caregiver out of sight. What can be done about this behavior? You may just have to take what moments of privacy you can get, unfortunately, even if it means installing a lock or childproof knob on the bathroom door for that brief respite. For longer reprieves, try interesting your loved one in a favorite TV show, a puzzle, or a task such as folding laundry, sorting socks, stacking magazines, or putting dishes away.

4. Complaining and accusing. "You're trying to poison me." "You keep me locked up." "You steal from me." "You're cruel to me." It can be quite upsetting to hear such accusations when you're essentially devoting your life to a person with Alzheimer's disease, but these remarks sometimes may be the thanks you get. Why? Because people with AD may be looking for some explanation, however irrational, for the unfairness of their condition. Confusion, frustration, and despair are fueling their venomous remarks, which you should in no way take personally, no matter how personal they might seem. Can they be stopped? Probably not, because by defending yourself you may only add fuel to their fire. Usually it's better just to ignore such remarks or be sympathetic to them by saying such things as "I know you're having a tough time, and I'm sorry."

5. Repeating the same remark, behavior, or question. "Five times in 5 minutes," said one caregiver of the number of times her father had asked who she was, and that's when she finally realized how sick he really was. People with AD may repeat more than just questions, however. They may repeat the same remark or expression or the same activity such as flipping a coin, shuffling cards, or pacing back and forth for hours. Experts theorize this is a way a person with AD may be trying to maintain some degree of predictability and order in a world that's becoming progressively more confusing and chaotic—small consolation for caregivers, however, who must endure such irritation. Sometimes repetitive behaviors can be curtailed if you can do something to make the person feel more secure—looking at old photo albums, for example, singing old songs, or simply hugging the person or giving a massage. It may also help to redirect a repetitive activity—going for a walk to visit someone, for example, to give a purpose to pacing. As for those questions that seem to have no end, resist announcing to your loved one the number of times you've already answered. You're better off just hoping your next time will be your last.

> *People with AD may repeat the same remark or expression or the same activity such as flipping a coin, shuffling cards, or pacing back and forth for hours.*

6. Stubbornness and defiance. "If my mother were a child of mine, she'd be spending a lot of time standing in the corner, that's for sure." That remark does a lot to sum up the way many caregivers feel in response to how defiant their loved ones can be. People with AD may resist being dressed and bathed, and they may refuse to eat at the proper times. As with many difficult behaviors associated with this disease, however, often fear and confusion are to blame. The person may feel threatened by even the most mundane activities of daily life, whether it's having his or her hair cut or teeth brushed. What may appear to be defiance also may simply be due to a lack of understanding. A command as simple as "Please sit down to dinner," for example, may not be well understood and hence not well obeyed. Try to be forgiving, and take paths of least resistance if your loved one seems purposely uncooperative. The person with AD may actually be doing the best he or she can.

7. Stealing. One caregiver reports that her husband one summer started coming home with armloads of sweet corn every afternoon, which wouldn't have been a problem if they had had a garden. But they didn't. Her husband's disease had negated his understanding of ownership, so their neighbors' sweet corn suddenly was his sweet corn, too. Stealing can be a common problem for people with Alzheimer's disease, and a sticky one when taking people with the illness shopping. Trying to explain to a security guard that a loved one is not a thief but simply suffering from an illness can result in feeling on very thin ice indeed. In truth, however, people with AD may simply forget they're in a store. To deal with this problem, carry with you a note from your loved one's doctor explaining the condition. This written explanation can make for a better argument to a security guard than your fumbled words and blushed face. Short of that, suggest your loved one push the shopping cart to occupy his or her hands, or sew pockets closed on coats. To prevent certain ends, it sometimes can help to prevent the means.

> *People with AD may resist being dressed and bathed, and they may refuse to eat at the proper times. As with many difficult behaviors associated with this disease, often fear and confusion are to blame.*

8. Sexual improprieties. Myths are more common than truths regarding sexual behaviors in people with AD. While it's true that people with the illness may forget they're inadequately dressed in certain situations or may be less than discreet about certain masturbatory desires, it's very rare for sexual urges to be directed inappropriately toward another person. Even in the seemingly unconscionable instance in which a father with Alzheimer's disease might make a sexual advance toward his daughter, it should be clear that the motivation would be far more likely to be due to a case of mistaken identity rather than anything more aberrant. For example, it's not uncommon for fathers with AD to mistake their grown daughters for their wives at a younger age—hence the seemingly "romantic" attraction. Any sexual behaviors that become problematic should be addressed, however. People exposed to them should be apprised of your loved one's condition, and the behaviors themselves should be prevented whenever possible. This latter tip doesn't mean scolding your loved one, because Alzheimer's has destroyed areas of the brain responsible for letting the person know he or she has even done anything wrong. Try instead to avoid situations in which such embarrassments might occur in the first place.

9. Physical aggression. People with Alzheimer's disease sometimes can become physically aggressive, especially in later stages of the disease, but, again, this behavior needs to be attributed to their illness more than intent. "My mom's thing was to kick," says one former caregiver, his mother now deceased. "And it wouldn't take much to get her going. After a while we realized it was just her way of expressing dissatisfaction she couldn't express in other way, but it still hurt." Caregivers need to realize that acts of physical aggression are motivated by frustration, fear, and confusion, not personal vendettas. The best way to prevent such outbursts is to try to create as peaceful an environment for your loved one as possible. If they do occur, do your best just to ignore them.

10. Delusional thinking. Normal neurological connections in the brain of people with AD can become so scrambled that past experiences—or fears of future experiences—can be confused with reality. The result, unfortunately, is that you could be accused of committing acts that someone else did to your loved one years ago. Or you could be accused of doing things that represent things your loved is afraid might happen in the future. This situation can be very frustrating as well as emotionally upsetting, but simply by helping your loved one feel safe and secure, you can help control these types of delusional thoughts.

Catastrophic Reactions: Don't Add More Thunder to the Storms

As we've described, people with Alzheimer's disease may suddenly "lose it" for no apparent reason and begin screaming, crying, cursing, throwing things, or even mounting a physical attack against others in

The World Through AD-Colored Glasses

In the years since Alzheimer's disease has begun to receive the attention it has, various authors have attempted to write about their own experiences with the disease, with surprising success. Some of these writers have talked about the fear that accompanies the mysterious onset of symptoms and the anger they have felt for being dealt such a cruel fate. More than any other sentiment, however, a feeling of profound loneliness seems to pervade these writings as the authors tell of what it's like to feel increasingly alienated, not just from their families and friends but from themselves.

Consider, for example, the words of Cary Henderson, a former history professor who writes in *Partial View: An Alzheimer's Journal,* "One of the worst things about Alzheimer's disease is that you're so alone with it. Nobody around you really knows what's going on . . . and most of the time we don't know what's going on ourselves."[15]

The loneliness theme emerges again in this account given by Larry Rose in his book *Show Me the Way Home:* "I have a sadness and anxiety that I have never experienced before. It feels like I am the only person in the world with this disease."[16]

In the hauntingly titled *Who Will I Be When I Die?* Christine Boden writes, "We know that something is terribly wrong with us. We seem to be losing touch with even who we are. We need all the help we can get."[17]

their presence. Just as suddenly as such a storm strikes, however, it can subside and leave its perpetrator with no memory that it ever occurred. What's going on?

To understand such "squalls," it can help to understand what Alzheimer's disease does to the brain. By destroying brain tissue responsible for making sense of incoming data, the disease can make the world of someone with AD a very confusing and scary place. As a result, people with AD can suffer from "information overload" very easily and begin to stress out in situations that for someone without the disease would be no problem at all. Too many people in a room, music that's too loud, an upsetting memory from the distant past, or even just a mild reprimand from a caregiver—they can't handle it and they react.

> *People with Alzheimer's disease may suddenly "lose it" for no apparent reason and begin screaming, crying, cursing, throwing things, or even mounting a physical attack against others.*

By why so dramatically? In addition to damaging parts of the brain responsible for handling stress, Alzheimer's opens the gates for the expression of this stress by destroying parts of the brain responsible for keeping things like fear, frustration, and anger in check. The area is called the *amygdala,* and it can begin to suffer fairly early in the disease process. Often it begins to deteriorate shortly after the memory center, in fact, so emotional torrents such as those described here may be something you'll need to deal with fairly soon, if you haven't already.

The best way to handle these outbursts? Try to avoid the situations apt to bring them on in the first place, some of which are listed in a moment. If one occurs, however, be as calm as possible and try to correct or remove the person from whatever circumstance might seem to be the cause. Do not make matters worse by scolding. The person's ability to listen to reason plummets to new lows during such eruptions. You're better off to express your love and to assure the person everything is all right. You will risk making these tempests only worse by adding thunder or lightening of your own.

Emotional outbursts known as catastrophic reactions may be prevented by protecting your loved one from the following situations:

- Needing to think about too many things at once
- Feeling treated like a child
- Feeling frustrated due to difficulty communicating

- Being tired or not feeling well
- Being confused by something seen or heard
- Being frustrated by not being able to do something
- Feeling anxious due to feeling inadequate
- Not understanding a request or command
- Being cared for by someone who is in a hurry or showing signs of being upset

A DAY IN THE LIFE OF SOMEONE WITH AD

What might a typical day with someone who has AD actually look like? This will depend on many factors, but experts from the Alzheimer's Association offer this schedule as a basic guide, nonetheless. You'll need to improvise on any schedule you establish as new situations arise, they concede, but it can be helpful to have at least a basic "theme" to work from. If nothing else, "a patterned day allows you to spend less time and energy trying to figure out what to do from moment to moment," they point out.

Morning:
- Get your loved one washed and dressed.
- Prepare and feed your loved one a healthful breakfast.
- Have your own breakfast as you engage your loved one in conversation.
- Go for a walk, do some chores around the house, read a book together, or watch a favorite show on TV.
- Spend some quiet time.
- Eat lunch.

Afternoon:
- Listen to music, do a crossword puzzle, or work on a craft.
- Take another walk, run some errands, or do more chores around the house or yard.

- Have a healthful snack.

- Have more quiet time or a nap.

Evening:

- Prepare and eat dinner.

- Clean up the kitchen.

- Play cards or an easy board game, give your loved one a massage, or watch TV or a video movie.

- Give your loved one a shower or bath, read a book or look at magazines, and get ready for bed.

A Word on Cigarettes and Alcohol: "Just Say No"

Should people with AD be allowed to continue to smoke or drink if either or both have been their custom over the years? For safety reasons, most experts say no. Smoking can be enough of a fire hazard even for the unimpaired, not to mention a health risk, but in the forgetful hands of someone with AD, it can be a recipe for disaster. The same goes for alcohol. It can dim the wits in all of us, but its effects can be even greater in people with dementias, putting them at even greater risk for lapses in judgment and falls. Fortunately, the "out of sight, out of mind" approach tends to work better in people with AD than those without the disease, so keep your fingers crossed that simply by not having cigarettes or alcohol around, your loved one may soon forget he or she ever had either habit at all. If this outcome proves not to occur, however, you may need to stand strong and "just say no" if and when your loved one requests to satisfy the urge.

SPECIAL THANKS TO CAREGIVERS

Caring for someone with AD can be a full-time job, all right—so much so, in fact, that cause for some long-overdue appreciation recently was acknowledged by researchers reporting in the *Journal of General Internal Medicine*. The researchers determined the cost of care currently being given to people with Alzheimer's by family members and friends—if the care were to be provided by paid professionals—totals over $18 billion a year![18] The U.S. economy owes AD caregivers a degree of gratitude commensurate with this colossal sum.

CHAPTER 5

Care for the Caregiver

❧

Respite is my number one need. I've been caring for my mom for
7 years and in that time have had one vacation lasting 3 days.

—*A CAREGIVER NEARING HER WIT'S END*

I f you saw the following job description, how might you react?

> **Wanted:** Someone to spend an average of 100 hours a week to over-
> see the physical and emotional well-being of another human being.
> Expect frustration, depression, rejection, occasional abuse, and
> chronic fatigue. No benefits, no vacation, no room for advancement,
> and no salary. (An annual fee, in fact, of approximately $12,500 may
> be required to cover the cost of goods and services not provided by
> the applicant.)

You'd probably assume the ad was some kind of joke, but it wouldn't
be. It would be an accurate description of what's required to be the primary caregiver of someone with Alzheimer's disease. "There's probably not a more challenging disease from the caregiver's standpoint,"
says Laura Gitlin, Ph.D., the director of Community Homecare Research at the College of Health Professions at Thomas Jefferson

University in Philadelphia. "Emotionally, physically, and even financially, the burdens of this illness on caregivers can be tremendous."

In a nationwide survey of over 1,500 caregivers done by the Alzheimer's Association in 1996, three-quarters of the respondents reported feeling depressed; nearly half said they weren't getting enough sleep; and they reported stress-related health problems, employment complications, and family conflicts more than caregivers of people with other diseases.[1] No wonder caregivers of people with Alzheimer's are sometimes called the "hidden" victims of this disease. For an illness not by definition contagious, AD sure can spread a lot of woe.

But help is available. As we'll be seeing in this chapter, the problems caregivers face are being studied as never before and solutions are being found. Organizations such as the Alzheimer's Association, the Alzheimer's Disease Education and Referral Center (ADEAR), the National Family Caregiver's Association (NFCA), and REACH (Resources for Enhancing Alzheimer's Caregiver Health) are looking at caregiver stress as a crisis and giving it the attention it deserves.

> *As powerless as you might sometimes feel, you are everything to your loved one and need to stay strong, accordingly.*

We'll be looking at ways you as a caregiver can get in the right kind of shape—emotionally as well as physically—to handle the challenges that lie ahead. We'll also look at the warning signs caregivers should look for that could indicate stress is becoming a problem. These concerns are very important, because *you* as a caregiver are very important. As powerless as you might sometimes feel, you are *everything* to your loved one and need to stay strong, accordingly, and take this chapter to heart with that point in mind.

GIFTS FOR THE GIVERS

Please keep something else in mind as you embark on what health experts acknowledge to be perhaps the greatest of all caregiving challenges: By giving, you as a caregiver also can receive. That fact might seem hard to believe given the picture we have of AD caregivers at their wit's end, but, if handled properly, caregiving can be a nourishing experience for caregiver and "care getter" alike. This isn't to say problems won't arise, because they will. The disease is simply too unpredictable to allow caregivers to prepare for the ever-changing behaviors they're likely to encounter. But as with all great challenges, great rewards are possible—and not just the obvious one of knowing we're improving the quality of life for another human being. As we witness the steady decline of some of life's most essential capacities in our loved ones, we can more deeply appreciate these capacities in ourselves.

*A*s we witness the steady decline of some of life's most essential capacities in our loved ones, we can more deeply appreciate these capacities in ourselves.

The ability to read a good book, to enjoy a great meal, to write a heart-felt letter, to engage in a thoughtful conversation, or even simply to love—these are abilities that we take for granted but that the person with AD loses a little more of every day. If we're able to savor these capacities more as our loved ones are able to enjoy them less, their struggles will not have been in vain, and their losses will have given us a very great gift indeed.

And the best way to appreciate these gifts fully? Not to feel depressed by your caregiving role but rather to feel stimulated by it. Much as a marathon runner needs to prepare mentally as well as physically for the challenge of those 26.2 miles, you as a caregiver will need to get in shape for the "marathon" that lies ahead of you—hence the importance of taking care of yourself in the ways that will be explained in this chapter. You will need to remain strong both physically and emotionally to meet this challenge, and your ability to do that is going to depend on basically four things: being well nourished, being in good physical condition, being well rested, and "being realistic," says Avrene Brandt, Ph.D., an expert in the area of caregiver stress and the author of *Caregiver's Reprieve.* "This can't be emphasized enough, because so often I see caregivers burn themselves out simply by failing to recognize that there's only so much one person can do for another. Caregiving is not about total self-sacrifice," Dr. Brandt says. "It's about learning to balance the patient's needs with the caregiver's needs, because this is the only way caregivers can sustain themselves."

CONTROL WHAT YOU CAN, NOT WHAT YOU CAN'T

Consider registered nurse Colleen Brooks, who, as the owner and chief operator of a small personal care facility for people with AD and other dementias, has had to learn to be realistic to make her living. "It can be hazardous duty, all right," she joked on a recent visit to her facility known as William's Manor in Wind Gap, Pennsylvania. "This morning I had applesauce spit in my face, yesterday I got kicked, and tomorrow who knows what I'll run into," she says. "I should probably wear shin guards and a helmet, I know, but this is just how this disease is, and you've got to accept it without taking it personally. There's not much chance of changing behavior like this, either, which is something else caregivers need to accept. You've just got to work at controlling what you can, things like comfort and safety, and not worry about what you can't."

> *You will need to remain strong both physically and emotionally to meet this challenge, and your ability to do that is going to depend on basically four things: being well nourished, being in good physical condition, being well rested, and being realistic.*

This is not a time for trying to be perfect or a control freak, in other words. "People with this disease usually can't be disciplined because they can't remember what they've been told," Brooks points out. "You're best off just trying to create the kind of secure and peaceful environment that's most likely to keep them from getting upset and acting out in the first place."

We'll be looking more at this aspect of caregiving in our next chapter, but the point to be made here is simply this: Don't be defeated by your own diligence. "Caregiver stress often is the result of people simply trying too hard, of wanting to change things that can't be changed, and of being in denial about the degree of impairment they're going to need to deal with," says Dr. Brandt. "Less often can be more in terms of caring for this disease. To reduce stress, we may simply need to recognize our limits."

STOPPING STRESS BEFORE IT STARTS

We need to recognize something else to keep from falling prey to the pitfalls of caregiver stress: the importance of stopping trouble even before it starts. "The old saying about an ounce of prevention being worth a pound of cure is certainly true," says Dr. Brandt. "In this case, it might even be worth a ton."

Check out these following stress-preventing strategies with that in mind. Or think of them as "training tips"—ways to "get in shape" for the challenge that lies ahead. Like that marathon runner, you're about to embark on a difficult journey, emotionally as well as physically, and it will help to be well prepared. Some of these strategies also can be helpful even if you notice signs of stress have already begun. Consider them not just preventive, therefore, but therapeutic as well.

Eat Well

Good nutrition is one of the most important bases caregivers need to cover to maintain physical as well as emotional stamina, yet it's an area they often neglect because of time constraints or lack of appetite due to stress. The result can be a major catch-22, unfortunately, as eating poorly can make caregivers even more vulnerable to the very stress that could be causing them to eat poorly in the first place. "There's no question that poor nutritional habits can deplete both our

Fish, the "Caregiver's Special"

If a single food could be considered a caregiver's best friend, it would have to be fish rich in the nutrient docosahexaenoic acid (DHA). Research suggests it may help AD caregivers by helping them combat depression and stress.

In one study reported in the *Journal of Clinical Investigation,* scientists from the Toyama Medical and Pharmaceutical University in Japan found that college students faced with the stress of preparing for exams were able to do so more calmly than a control group after being given 1.5 to 1.8 grams of DHA daily for 3 months. The difference in stress levels between the two groups, as measured by acts of aggression, in some cases was as great as 46 percent. Lead researcher of the study, Tomohito Hamazaki, speculates that this calming effect of DHA may help explain why it also appears to help protect against heart disease.[2]

In addition to keeping stress down, DHA may help caregivers keep their spirits up. Research by Joseph R. Hibbeln, M.D., of the National Institutes of Health has found that as levels of fish consumption go up in countries around the world, rates of depression come down. In Japan, for example, where fish consumption is the highest in the world at 140 pounds per person a year, rates of depression are the lowest in the world at a scant 0.12 percent. In New Zealand, by comparison, where the annual fish consumption is only

emotional as well as physical reserves, especially as we age," says Jane Townsend, R.D., the nutritional care planner at the Phoebe Home for the aged in Allentown, Pennsylvania. "Skipping meals, for example, constitutes an immediate stress to the body by driving blood sugar levels down, and failing to get adequate nutrients in the long run can whittle away at physical and emotional endurance alike," Townsend says. Don't subject yourself to these needless drawbacks. Eat at least three nutritious meals a day that include plenty of fresh fruits and

25 pounds per person, rates of depression are a precipitous 5.8 percent. In the United States, levels fall somewhere in between: a per capita consumption of 50 pounds of fish per year and a depression rate of approximately 3 percent.[3] Other studies have shown that depressed people tend to have low levels of DHA in their blood, thus adding more evidence to the connection.[4]

Why should DHA have this effect? "Evidence suggests DHA helps regulate serotonin, a neurotransmitter known for its 'feel-good' qualities," explains Jean Carper in *Your Miracle Brain.* Check out these best sources of DHA with that observation in mind.[5]

Fish (3½ ounces, canned or raw)	DHA, in grams
Mackerel	1.4
Herring	1.0
Sardines	1.0
Anchovies	0.9
Sablefish	0.9
Tuna, bluefin	0.9
Whitefish	0.9
Bluefish	0.8
Salmon	0.8
Lake trout	0.5

vegetables, fish, lean meats, beans, and whole-grain foods rich in fiber for healthy digestion. Don't hesitate to indulge in healthful between-meal snacks to keep your energy and spirits up.

Keep In Good Shape

Exercise might seem like the last thing you should have to worry about as a caregiver, yet it can be an important ally, says Jamie Clark, the president of the American Senior Fitness Association in New Smyrna, Florida. Not only is exercise a proven stress reducer and spirit booster, but "keeping physically fit can help caregivers avoid the exhaustion their duties can cause, and this is true of aerobic exercise, in particular," Clark notes. This benefit is especially valuable in the later stages of Alzheimer's disease when some people with the illness may need considerable help getting around, she says.

As for whether the caregiver should include the person with AD in exercise efforts, this matter needs to be a personal decision based on the condition and willingness of the person with AD, Clark says. The advantage to including the person with Alzheimer's is that exercise can help ward off many of the physical disabilities as well as help temper the physical aggression that can make some people with AD particularly difficult to manage. On the downside, however, a caregiver's time for privacy may be lost. As a kind of compromise, caregivers might try working out with their loved ones to an exercise video or daily exercise program on TV that meets both people's needs, Clark says. At least 20 to 30 minutes of aerobic exercise daily such as walking, cycling, swimming, or doing yard work, supplemented by light stretching and possibly several weight-training sessions a week, should be a caregiver's goal (see sidebar, "It Can Be a Workout"). If you're the type who enjoys company, check out fitness programs offered at your local YMCA, community college, or health club.

Get Enough Rest

This recommendation might sound like the impossible dream, but with some imagination and perhaps a touch of tolerance, it can be done, say Nancy Mace, M.A., and Peter Rabins, M.D., authors of the caregivers' guide, *The 36-Hour Day*. It might mean learning to catch a quick nap in the afternoon when your loved one might also be resting or perhaps simply being more accepting of behaviors that might otherwise cause you to lose sleep, these experts say. If Grandpa likes to get up in the middle of the night and sit on the couch, for example, let him. As long as he's content and safe, there's no reason you should have to lose sleep watching him. It also can be helpful to keep people with AD active during the day, so they'll be genuinely fatigued when bedtime comes, Mace and Rabins say. As a last resort, consider allowing your loved one to be prescribed a medication to aid sleep, especially if late-night wandering becomes a problem. These medications need to be used with care, because they can present dangers for people with AD, but for caregiver and care getter alike, sleep medications can be well worth it if adequate rest is the result.[6]

Be Patient

Just as Rome wasn't built in a day, caregivers shouldn't think they can solve the problems of caregiving overnight. Trying to do too much too fast could prevent you from accomplishing much of anything, in fact, so it's important to be patient and go slowly. "If you're at the end of your rope, single out one thing that you can change to make life easier and work on that," Mace and Rabins say. Start with the most basic challenges first, such as bathing, eating, and dressing, which for many people with AD can actually cause the most trouble. Once at least some modicum of normalcy has been established by solving these problems, you'll have a foundation to work from as you move on to others.[7]

> *Start with the most basic challenges first, such as bathing, eating, and dressing, which for many people with AD can actually cause the most trouble.*

Be Honest

It might not be the easiest policy, but it's the best—honesty with your loved one, honesty with your friends and family, and honesty with yourself. With your loved one, be honest about what you're feeling so you can work together as a team, and ask your loved one to be open with you in return so there can be a foundation of trust to help things go more smoothly as the disease grows worse. With family members or friends, be honest about what kind of help you need, how much, and when. And with yourself, be

It Can Be a Workout

Several times a day Myra needs to help her mother in and out of bed, up and out of chairs, to and from the bathroom, and up and down the stairs. Assisting her mom in and out of the car and the shower are other regular duties, as is helping her off the floor, unfortunately, when she takes one of her all-too-frequent spills. It's a lot of work for someone of any age, especially for Myra, who, in addition to having high blood pressure, diabetes, and arthritis, is 75.

"It's getting to be a significant problem, and especially as more and more elderly people are finding themselves in the caregiving role," says Laura Gitlin, Ph.D., who, along with several other researchers from an organization known as REACH (Resources for Enhancing Alzheimer's Caregiver Health), recently studied the dangers older caregivers face. Injuries to the lower back, neck, and knees were found to be the most common complaints, but emotional stress and fatigue in general were found to be prevalent, as well.

As a result of their study, these researchers compiled a list of the following six questions that can help caregivers determine whether their caregiving duties may be posing undue risks.

honest about when you've reached your limits so you can get whatever counseling you might need to keep you from breaking down. "There's no sense in being a martyr with this illness because that becomes a lose-lose for everybody," says Penny Martin, R.N., a research coordinator on caregiver stress for the Philadelphia Geriatric Center. "Caregivers need to recognize their limits, and without feelings of guilt."

Be Flexible

Because the very nature of Alzheimer's disease entails unpredictability, caregivers can save themselves a lot of trouble by learning to be

1. Have you experienced back pain in the past 3 months while helping your loved one?

2. Are you worried you might hurt your back by helping your loved one?

3. Are you concerned you might hurt your loved one by attempting to give assistance?

4. Have you or your loved one experienced problems with balance in your day-to-day maneuverings?

5. Has either of you experienced a fall in the past 6 months?

6. Do you or your loved one have any other health problems that worry you?

Any caregiver who answers yes to one or more of these questions has legitimate cause for concern, Dr. Gitlin says, and should look into getting help from a physical therapist who, with even one visit to the home, can give valuable instruction on making the physical demands of caregiving as stress-free as possible.

tolerant and "going with the flow," the experts say. Trying to impose too much discipline and order can be an exercise in futility," says nurse Brooks. "Besides, there's a limited amount you can do to discipline [people] with Alzheimer's because they can't remember what you've told them," she points out. "Rather than make rules you can't enforce, it's usually easier just not to make any rules at all." This tip doesn't mean allowing total anarchy, but it does mean learning to accommodate rather than scold, especially since the scolding may produce just the opposite of its intended effect. "Many people with this illness are emotionally very fragile and may react to even mild reprimand by becoming quite upset," Brooks explains. Caregivers need to learn what's worth worrying about and what's not, she says. "If Dad wants to wear his army uniform one day, let him. Only behaviors that risk the patient's safety need to be worried about."

Be Knowledgeable

Taking care of someone with Alzheimer's disease is no different from any other endeavor in that the more you know, the better you're going to do. This was shown in a recent study supported by the National Institute of Nursing Research (NINR) in which caregivers who had participated in a 14-hour caregiver-training course reported having an easier time caring for their loved ones than a group of caregivers who had not taken the course. The results of this study should be considered especially important in light of other research that shows that people with AD whose needs are not well understood are more apt to become physically aggressive. Better care can make for better behavior, in other words, and hence a better quality of life for both the caregiver and care getter.[8]

> Caregivers can save themselves a lot of trouble by learning to be tolerant and "going with the flow."

Be Selfish

This means taking time to do what *you* want to do and not feeling guilty about it. How well you take care of yourself is going to be reflected in how well you're going to be able to take care of your loved one, so consider your self-indulgences time well spent. "I love my husband dearly," says Marianne, "but on the days I take him to his day care center for a couple of hours, I feel free. It's my favorite time of the week, and I think it's good for him, too, because he usually comes home in a better mood." You might feel you're being selfish to take time for things you like to do, but you *shouldn't*, the experts agree. Consider it money in the bank, an investment that will produce considerable "interest" in the form of renewed energy and enthusiasm for your caregiving duties.

Be an Imperfectionist

If you're a person who finds comfort in precision, order, neatness, and control, be prepared to lower your standards when caring for someone with AD. Because the mental world of people with AD can be in disarray, so can their outer world as reflected by their dress, personal neatness, and manners of eating. Depending on the person and the stage of the illness, you may need to endure table manners no tidier than those of a toddler and clothing preferences akin to those of a circus clown. "These behaviors are the inevitable consequences of AD's march across the human brain," says John Medina, Ph.D., a professor of molecular biology at the University of Washington School of Medicine and author of *What You Need to Know About Alzheimer's Disease.*[9] In the later stages of AD, people may need assistance even in the bathroom, so the squeamish should beware.

> *You might feel you're being selfish to take time for things you like to do, but you shouldn't, the experts agree.*

Be a Journalist

According to Plato, "the life which is unexamined is not worth living." We won't go that far, but we will say that keeping a written account of your experiences as a caregiver can be a great stress reducer in addition to helping you find the best ways to do your job. "Writing can let you vent emotions you might not otherwise have an outlet to express," says Daniel Kuhn, M.S.W., the director of education at the Mather Institute on Aging in Evanston, Illinois. From a more practical standpoint, keeping a journal may help you see patterns that could be useful in determining how to manage your loved one in the future, Kuhn says. He offers these tips for improving your chances of success:

- Don't intimidate yourself by thinking this journal has to be a great work of art or that it has to be grammatically correct. This is your private project that no one else has to see.

- Use whatever means is most convenient. If you have access to a computer and enjoy using it, fine. Otherwise a good old-fashioned typewriter or even just pencil and paper can get the same job done.

- Be totally uninhibited and say whatever comes to mind. This is your time to vent, an intellectual approach to the primal scream.

- Try to make an entry in your journal every day, but don't force yourself. The goal of your journal is to reduce stress, remember, not create even more of it.

Be Willing to Laugh

"Without a sense of humor, I'd have been a goner long ago," jokes Helen, whose husband is now in the middle stages of AD. "It's either laugh or cry sometimes, and the laughing is a lot more fun. I thinks it's good for my husband, too." Research over the years has come up with plenty of evidence to support the kind of medicinal mirth Helen is talking about. The positive emotions associated with a good laugh have been shown to boost the body's immune system, help reduce stress, and possibly even help protect against heart disease. As comedian Bill Cosby has wisely observed, "If you can find humor in something, you can survive it." (See "Humor Can Be Serious Medicine" later in this chapter.)

TWELVE SIGNS OF CAREGIVER STRESS AND WHAT TO DO ABOUT THEM

Even our most diligent efforts to insulate ourselves against caregiver stress can allow some of the stuff to leak through, and we need to be aware of when this happens. Learning to manage stress in this sense is a lot like learning to manage our cars: preventive maintenance is key. Just as responding to warning signs such as blinking oil lights and squeaky fan belts can keep our cars from breaking down, responding to certain stress signals from our bodies can keep *us* from breaking down.

According to the Alzheimer's Association, the kinds of "blinking lights" described here can help caregivers know ahead of time that trouble, in the form of an emotional breakdown or physical illness, could be on the way. If you notice any of these signs in yourself or in anyone else involved with your loved one's care, call your doctor or the Alzheimer's Association and ask about how to get help. Psychological counseling often can be beneficial, as can attending a caregiver support group or participating in a caregiver's training class (see the appendix). Getting help with the actual day-to-day duties of caregiving also can be a great stress reliever, so consider this as an option, too. As explained in more detail in the next chapter, many services are now available give caregivers the help they need inside as well as outside the home.

> *Even our most diligent efforts to insulate ourselves against caregiver stress can allow some of the stuff to leak through, and we need to be aware of when this happens.*

Whatever you do, do not just assume that exasperation is par for the caregiving course. It should not be. Caregiving always will present challenges, but they should not be overwhelming ones. If you feel yourself beginning to buckle under the weight, you owe it to yourself *and to your loved one* to get help. "To give care, we sometimes need to receive care, and we shouldn't feel the least bit demeaned by it," Dr. Brandt says.

1. Denial. ("Dad's going to get over this. It's just going to take time.") The hardest part of Alzheimer's disease for many caregivers is accepting that their loved one is not going to get better. It's easier to care for someone when there's hope for recovery, but caregivers of people with AD don't yet have this luxury. What caregivers often do instead, therefore, is to reach for the next best thing, and that's denial. "Denial is a very natural human reaction and can help us get through particularly tough situations until we're feeling strong enough to accept things as they really are," says Dr. Brandt. "But denial also can have distinct disadvantages if we allow it to continue too long. By sheltering us from the truth, denial can make the truth even more painful when it finally arrives." In the case of Alzheimer's disease, denial also can keep caregivers from properly managing an illness that's already difficult enough to manage as it is, Dr. Brandt says. "Caregivers need to know as much about this illness as they can in order to deal with it as best they can, and denial prevents that."

> *In the case of Alzheimer's disease, denial also can keep caregivers from properly managing an illness that's already difficult enough to manage as it is.*

2. Anger. ("If Mom asks that question one more time, I'm going to strangle her.") Anger can be another natural reaction to the seeming cruelty and injustice of Alzheimer's disease, but still an unhealthy one that risks doing more harm than good. Anger may be directed at the person with AD out of sheer frustration, or at the medical world for not having found a cure, or at friends or relatives for not better understanding the caregiver's plight. "Anger may even be motivated by a feeling of disappointment that a once-dignified and respected loved one has been reduced to such an unfortunate state," Dr. Brandt says. Whatever its reasons, anger risks adding insult to injury by making caregivers feel *guilty* for the anger they feel, thus driving their stress to an even higher level. This represents a potentially dangerous situation that needs to be addressed as quickly as possible, Dr. Brandt says. Physical abuse of people with AD by their caregivers is rare, but it does happen.

3. Social withdrawal. ("Dad needs me more than that stupid bowling team, and my game has been so bad anyway.") Again, dangerous thinking. If you've been heading in this direction, stop and make a U-turn or at least a very hard left. "By depriving themselves of outside stimulation, caregivers risk not just becoming resentful and depressed; they risk becoming less effective at the very duties they want to succeed at most," says Dr. Brandt. "The activity itself doesn't matter, just so long as it provides a sense of release and breaks the normal caregiving routine."

4. Anxiety. ("What's going to happen when Mom gets worse? I'm being stretched to my limit as it is.") A certain amount of anxiety is both natural and necessary because it can help motivate us to take needed actions. But too much anxiety can stymie the very decision-making processes needed to find solutions. If you find yourself feeling "There's just no way out of this," you need help. Consider joining a support group or using an adult day care center. Caregiver-training sessions also are available, as is help via the computer. No longer is Alzheimer's an unrecognized problem. The seriousness of this disease has aroused serious attention, and the benefits of that attention are now available in many forms.

> *A certain amount of anxiety is both natural and necessary because it can help motivate us to take needed actions. But too much anxiety can stymie the very decision-making processes needed to find solutions.*

5. Depression. ("I just don't care anymore. This is hopeless and so am I.") Depression is a frame of mind that can exist at many levels before it qualifies as clinical, and the sooner these lesser stages are dealt with, the better. "It's to be expected for caregivers to feel saddened by their situation, but it's more serious if there's a general feeling that life itself no longer matters," Dr. Brandt says. If you find this becoming the case, counseling could be needed. Even if your sadness does turn out to be clinical depression, the condition can effectively be treated with medications, counseling, or a combination of both. (For more on depression, see sidebar "How Sad Is Too Sad?")

6. Fatigue. ("Somehow it feels like I'm dragging a ball and chain around in everything I do.") Fatigue is like sadness in that a certain amount is to be expected. But fatigue that begins to pervade every aspect of your life is not. Be concerned if you seem to lack the energy for activities that were once enjoyable for you, or you find you're having trouble staying awake at critical times such as at work or while driving. You may need to adjust your caregiving schedule or get additional

How Sad Is Too Sad?

Depression can be like that noise coming from our refrigerators in that we can become so accustomed to it, we fail to recognize it even exists. It's vitally important not to let this happen with depression, however, because in addition to being a burden for you, depression can be yet another straw on the already-burdened back of your loved one. "A dangerously vicious cycle can develop where the depression of the caregiver feeds the depression of the patient and vice versa," says Ronald Podell, M.D., a psychotherapist and the codirector of the Westbridge Psychiatric Medical Group in Los Angeles. "The person with AD isn't usually able to take the lead and get help, of course, so it's the duty of the caregiver to break this type of cycle."

Here are symptoms to watch for that could indicate your sadness has reached a point where professional help should be sought. Two

help. Taking time to squeeze some exercise into your day also can help fight fatigue, believe it or not, as can eating well, as explained later.

7. Trouble sleeping. ("How can I sleep when I never know when George is going to want to get up and start dancing to the stereo?") Even if the time does become available for caregivers to sleep, sleep can be difficult because of anxieties associated with their caregiving duties. If you're having a problem sleeping because of your loved one's nocturnal activities, talk to your loved one's doctor about a medication that might help with the sleep problems your loved one is having. Or consider an herbal remedy. Frena Gray-Davidson, who conducts workshops and training sessions for Alzheimer's caregivers, reports that diffusing the essential oil of lavender throughout a bedroom can be helpful as a sleep aid for people with Alzheimer's disease and other dementias.[10] If you're still having trouble sleeping once your loved one has been made more restful, see your doctor. Counselor more of these symptoms experienced for more than about 2 weeks should be cause for concern:

- A loss of interest in formerly enjoyable activities
- Chronic feelings of agitation
- Lack of energy
- Feelings of guilt
- Feelings of worthlessness
- Difficulty concentrating or making decisions
- Unusual gains or losses in weight
- Thoughts that you might be better off dead

ing could help, as could a sleep medication or some lavender oil of your own.

8. Irritability. ("I found myself shouting obscenities at Mom the other day, and then I even gave the pizza delivery guy a hard time. I'm just not myself.") As with the other signs of caregiver stress, irritability is understandable, but it's still a sign that your body and mind are in a state of unhealthful unrest. Try to identify the aspects of your caregiving that you're finding the most bothersome, and make efforts to correct them. If certain behaviors by your loved one are fueling your irritation, work on those in particular. Do *not* assume that your only recourse is to remain an ill-tempered wretch, because that's apt to only make matters worse by further upsetting your loved one. Do yourselves both a favor and get some help, through counseling, a support group, or a service to lighten the load of your daily caregiving duties.

9. Lack of concentration. ("I'm getting forgetful just like Grandpa.") Paradoxical but true. Caregivers can become so overwhelmed by their unrelenting responsibilities that they can begin to experience some of the same confusion as their loved ones. The brain simply cannot function at full capacity when overloaded with physical and emotional stress. If you experience difficulty concentrating, you're going to have to make some changes or get some help. Caregiving is simply too challenging an endeavor to handle in a mental fog. Quick decisions can be required, plus attention to details such as medication schedules. It's not a job to be tackled with anything less than all of our "cards" neatly stacked.

As with the other signs of caregiver stress, irritability is understandable, but it's still a sign that your body and mind are in a state of unhealthful unrest.

10. Substance abuse. ("More and more I'm finding I need a couple of drinks to help me cope.") This is not an uncommon reaction to the stresses of caregiving, but it is a dangerous one. In addition to risking addiction and consequent health problems, heavy drinking—or substance abuse of any kind, for that matter—can impair the ability to function competently as a caregiver. If you're not sure whether your level of indulgence has crossed the line and become problematic, ask yourself the simple question of whether it's begun to interfere with your work—your caregiving included. If your honest answer is yes, talk to your doctor. The longer you continue to escape the stresses of caregiving this way, the greater the health risks will be for you and your loved one alike.

11. Eating irregularities. ("Sometimes I just want to eat potato chips all day, and other times I don't want to eat at all.") Periods of eating too much followed by periods of eating too little are signs of emotional turmoil, and they should be addressed for physical as well as psychological reasons. By overeating, caregivers risk burdening themselves with guilt; by undereating, they risk irritability and physical weakness, Dr. Brandt says. If meals are a problem, consider getting outside help. The Alzheimer's Association can put you in touch with a service that can provide meals on a regular basis, but if not even this strategy helps you eat on a regular schedule, you might want to consider psychological counseling as the next step. Eating disorders can be serious business, capable of doing both physical and emotional damage.

12. Health problems. ("I can't even remember the last time I felt well.") This would seem to be the most obvious sign of caregiver stress, but often it's overlooked as caregivers fail to attribute their health problems to the proper source. Our minds and bodies are intimately linked, however, so what stresses one will stress the other, and

> *High levels of stress can increase risks for headaches, digestive problems, high blood pressure, and possibly even more serious conditions such as heart disease and even cancer.*

caregivers need to keep this well in mind. High levels of stress can increase risks for headaches, digestive problems, high blood pressure, and possibly even more serious conditions such as heart disease and even cancer, so don't risk it. If you find yourself experiencing an increase in health problems, see your doctor and explain the pressures you're under. You may be a candidate for counseling to help put your mind—and thus your body—more at ease.

HUMOR CAN BE SERIOUS MEDICINE

We don't usually think of Abraham Lincoln as much of a chucklemeister, but even he appreciated the value of humor as evidenced by these words he once delivered to his cabinet: "Why don't you laugh, gentlemen? With the grave situations that are upon me day and night, if I did not laugh I should die. You need the medicine as much as I do."

Lincoln was more than a little prescient in making that remark. In studies done recently at Loma Linda University in California, researchers have found that laughter appears to activate key elements of

Edicts from the Experienced

In our discussions with dozens of people in researching this book, we often were impressed with sage advice, interesting remarks, and otherwise illuminating observations made not by health experts but rather by caregivers themselves—"experts" graduated from the school of hard knocks. Experience is often our best teacher, after all, and with Alzheimer's, there's always something new to be learned. Here are some of the caregivers' bits of wisdom that we found most worthy of being shared:

"When something goes wrong, it only makes things worse to get upset about it. I just try to learn from it instead."

"You can't go trying to impose reality on someone with this disease. You're better off just going along with theirs."

"There's a lot that can be very funny about this disease, if we can just learn to look at it that way. Last summer at a neighbor's picnic, we looked over and there was my husband in his underwear playing in the kiddie pool. We never laughed so hard in all our lives."

"I've learned to be careful about assuming Mom doesn't know when we're talking about her. People with this disease can be more aware than they sometimes appear."

"I've learned to expect the unexpected and then still be surprised."

"My support group has been wonderful. It helps me know I'm not alone."

"I think it's important to involve your loved as much as possible in what's going on. I tell my husband everything I can about his condition, which let's us work together against it as a team."

the immune system such as T lymphocytes, gamma interferon, and immunoglobin A—the microscopic soldiers that defend us against maladies ranging from colds to cancer.[11] Laughter also appears to help protect us from the ravages of stress by reducing the hormone epinephrine, which can elevate heart rate and blood pressure while also *suppressing* the activity of the immune system.

Might these mechanisms help explain another discovery by scientists from the University of Michigan at Ann Arbor that pessimists tend to suffer from more health problems than optimists?[12] And might they have played a role in the miraculous recovery of former *Saturday Review* editor Norman Cousins, who back in the mid-1960s seemingly cured himself from a terminal illness by watching funny movies all day?[13]

Researchers are beginning to think so. "What is clear is that the worse you feel about yourself and the worse your outlook on life, the worse your health may be," write Francis Brennan, Ph.D., and Carl Charnetski, Ph.D., in *Feeling Good Is Good for You: How Pleasure Can Boost Your Immune System and Lengthen Your Life.*[14] By keeping our spirits up, in other words, we may be able to keep our health up, too. It's certainly worth a try.

A Green Light to Laugh

But what's funny about Alzheimer's disease?

Nothing, which is precisely why humor can be so helpful in dealing with it. Humor has a unique power to brighten even the darkest situation, making it a medicine especially well suited for dealing with Alzheimer's disease.

But doesn't humor trivialize a loved one's condition? The very fact that someone might be concerned about that point argues that it does not. Some of the greatest humorists, after all, have made the funniest jokes about the people they have respected most.

So if you feel an urge to chuckle, or even just let go a toothy grin in response to a situation that strikes you as funny, don't hold back.

Humor is a great stress reducer and health booster, and it can help lift the spirits of your loved one, too.

TIPS FOR BREAKING THE SADNESS "HABIT"

While it's healthy to express the way you feel, especially when you're feeling sad, it's not healthy to feel sad for very long. As mentioned earlier, sadness that lasts more than about 2 weeks could be a sign of clinical depression, which could have serious consequences for both you and your loved one and should be treated by a doctor. Prolonged sadness also can begin to depress the body's immune system, increasing chances for physical illness. Some research suggests that even just brief periods of sadness also can compromise the immune system, so it's going to be important for you as a caregiver to keep your chin up as much as possible.

Humor is a great stress reducer and health booster, and it can help lift the spirits of your loved one, too.

But how can you do that when there's just not that much to be chipper about? Researchers are finding that we may have more control over this seemingly elusive state called happiness than we realize. While we tend to think of happiness as something that has to come to us, more often it's something we simply have to *go and get*.

Two pioneers in this way of thinking, Francis Brennan and Carl Charnetski, note in *Feeling Good Is Good for You*, "If you force yourself to act in ways that are out of sync with how you actually feel, your brain will change your attitude to come into accordance with your behavior."[15] That statement might sound like wishful thinking, but we certainly owe it to ourselves to try. What do we have to lose, after all, other than perhaps our blues? Drs. Brennan and Charnetski offer the following as instant mirth makers well worth a try:

- **Simply smile more.** Sounds easy enough, right? The simple act of smiling encourages our feelings to follow, these experts say. "The nerves connected to the face's smile muscles project right into the parts of the brain that help determine mood," they report. Simply by expressing happiness, therefore, "you send a signal to your brain that you are happy and voilà! You're happy."[16]

- **Put the cart before the horse.** Often the first step toward feeling happier is the hardest, because periods of sadness can create their own kind of inertia that can be difficult to be overcome. Just do it, Drs. Brennan and Charnetski say. Even if you're not in the mood to go out to dinner or to a movie or to visit a friend, do it anyway and you're likely to feel better simply for having made the effort.

- **Dwell on the positive.** Even if 90 percent of your life is a shambles and out of control, that leaves 10 percent that's not. So focus on this 10 percent 90 percent of the time, these doctors say. It's amazing how the other 90 percent will tend to disappear.

- **Act more; mope less.** Often we feel anxious or sad simply because we're dreading something we know we have to do. Again, just do it, these doctors advise. Even if the task turns out to be as unpleasant as we feared, it will haunt us no more.

- **Hang out with the right crowd.** The saying about misery loving company is true, so find some company that doesn't have any time for the stuff. This doesn't mean avoiding other caregivers and learning from them, but it does mean supplementing this company. Try to spend at least some time with people who are positive, energetic, and upbeat to entice you to be the same.

- **Vent.** This is where joining a caregiver support group can be helpful. To let happiness in, it can help to let anger and sadness out, so join a group of sympathetic listeners and do just that.

IN SUPPORT OF SUPPORT GROUPS

Why take precious time to be around others with the same problems as yours when you could be doing something else more enjoyable?

The central philosophy of support groups is that several heads can be better than one when it comes gaining perspective and solving problems, and thousands of caregivers worldwide currently are finding their participation in these groups extremely helpful. "I was never the group type but have been amazed at how much I get out of it," said one caregiver we talked to. "We talk about every possible aspect of what caregiving can involve, and the meetings give us a chance to sh are how we feel."

The central philosophy of support groups is that several heads can be better than one when it comes to gaining perspective and solving problems.

Indeed, the meetings leave no stones unturned as issues ranging from handling behavioral problems to finding reliable and affordable help are discussed. Even matters such as those regarding legal and financial aspects of AD get addressed periodically, and all free of charge. The groups generally consist of eight to 20 participants and are led either by a trained health care professional or fellow caregiver particularly experienced in Alzheimer's care. Meetings typically are held monthly, last about 2 hours, and are conducted in an informal, speak-as-needed style, and they can be discontinued by participants at any time. According to the Alzheimer's Association, these group meetings can help caregivers in the following ways:

- They can provide an outlet for emotions.

- They can minimize feelings of helplessness and isolation.

- They can help boost feelings of self-worth.

- They allow participants to share valuable knowledge and insights learned through experience.

- They allow participants to learn about resources available for helping them with their caregiving duties.

- They can provide a valuable respite from the stress of providing continual Alzheimer's care.

To locate a support group in your area, call the Alzheimer's Association's help line at (800) 272-3900, or check with a hospital or social service agency near you. For caregivers unable or unwilling to attend group meetings in person, help and information can still be obtained either by calling the Alzheimer's Association or by contacting its Web site at www.alz.com. The interactive quality of the group sessions will be lost this way, but there are other options for experiencing this quality, too. Caregivers can participate in a worldwide chat room online via e-mail by contacting the Alzheimer's Disease Research Center at Washington University in St. Louis ([314] 362-2882). For more information on how to join this informative group, see "Internet Resources" in the appendix. Similar groups devoted to assisting AD caregivers also are available through Internet providers such as America Online, CompuServe, Prodigy Internet, and the Microsoft Network. We should see this high number and variety of resources as a testimony to just how widespread a problem AD has become but also, more important, to the incredible amount of interest there is to provide help.

EMOTIONS TO EXPECT

Because the behaviors caused by Alzheimer's disease can be so diverse, so, too, can the emotional reactions it arouses in caregivers. These emotions can range from such expected ones as sadness and frustration to such unexpected ones as resentment, jealousy, anger, and even rage. This can be very surprising and even upsetting for caregivers because it can make them doubt their inherent kindness, yet the emotions are natural human reactions that caregivers need to understand so they can best deal with them, Dr. Brandt says.

> *Because the behaviors caused by Alzheimer's disease can be so diverse, so, too, can the emotional reactions it arouses in caregivers.*

Here are the feelings Dr. Brandt says caregivers should be prepared to experience, and possibly quite strongly. Not all caregivers will have all these reactions because every situation is so different, Dr. Brandt adds, but it can be helpful for caregivers to be prepared nonetheless.

Fear. This emotion usually is a caregiver's first response to learning a loved one has AD and an understandable one representing acute anxiety over a situation that poses a major threat to one's well-being or that of a loved one. Often this fear will be accompanied by confusion over an immediate course of action to take, but usually it gives over fairly soon to a form of self-protection known as denial.

Denial. Another normal reaction to news of AD, denial serves as a temporary period of escape from the reality of what's at hand, which can be a good thing by providing temporary shelter until a person feels ready to handle the truth. It can create problems, however, if allowed to continue too long.

> *Rarely is the caregiver rewarded with progress but instead experiences decline and often even considerable resistance.*

Anxiety. As denial gradually moves out, anxiety can begin to move in—anxiety about the future of you and your loved one alike. For a while this anxiety may be paralyzing, but it, too, eventually subsides as resources rooted in basic survival start to take hold and the caregiver digs in to cope.

Frustration. These coping efforts may result in frustration, as the seeming futilities of caregiving begin to mount. Rarely is the caregiver rewarded with progress but instead experiences decline and often even considerable resistance. The entire situation can suddenly seem almost maliciously absurd.

Resentment. Next may come the logical consequence of such exasperation: resentment—resentment for feeling trapped, resentment of other family members for not being more involved, resentment of the medical establishment for not having a better handle on this disease that is stealing away your life, and so forth.

Meet a Caregiver's Best Friend:
The Alzheimer's Association

You've noticed us mentioning the Alzheimer's Association repeatedly throughout this book, and for good reason: No other organization can offer so much, in so many ways, to so many people affected by this disease. Founded by family members of people with AD in 1980, the organization is the largest volunteer effort of its kind in the United States with approximately 200 chapters nationwide. Its mission: not just to help caregivers and patients learn about and manage Alzheimer's disease but also to raise funds for AD research to find better treatments, better diagnostic techniques, and a cure. The organization has raised more than $100 million for research since its inception, while its educational efforts include several newsletters, free educational brochures, and a toll-free help line. Call anytime during normal business hours, and you'll get a real person who will help answer virtually any question you might have. Whether it's a medical concern or you simply want information on how to find a physician, a counselor, a support group, a health care facility, or an attorney specializing in Alzheimer's issues, you'll have gone to the right place. To contact the Alzheimer's Association during business hours, call (800) 272-3900, or check out its Web site anytime at www.alz.org. You can even e-mail questions to info@alz.org. However you choose to contact the Alzheimer's Association, don't fail to do so. It's a resource not to be missed.

Anger. Then the shocker—resentment so strong it turns to anger. The anger comes from feeling wronged, from feeling helpless, from feeling annoyed, and from feeling unappreciated or even rebuffed by the person being cared for. Anger at someone so impaired is unacceptable, however, so it causes yet another unexpected emotion—guilt.

Guilt. Guilt is the emotional spanking caregivers give themselves for feeling anger toward someone so helpless, and it, too, can have negative consequences by eroding feelings of self-worth. Sometimes caregivers will try to compensate and become overly coddling of their loved one, but still the caregiver's self-esteem has been dealt a serious blow.

Feelings of isolation. With wounded self-esteem, the caregiver may now be reluctant to maintain outside social contacts and begin to suffer from loneliness, a loneliness compounded by the dwindling lines of communication with his or her loved one.

REACH to the Rescue

The hazards of being an AD caregiver have been well recognized and currently are the subject of intense study by an organization known as REACH (Resources for Enhancing Alzheimer's Caregiver Health). Formed in 1995 by the National Institutes of Health, the National Institute on Aging, and the National Institute of Nursing Research, the goal of REACH is to alleviate the problems that caregivers of people with AD face. "We're doing the best we can to help caregivers in every way possible, and it's important we do because the well-being of caregivers and their loved ones alike are at stake," says Laura Gitlin, Ph.D., the director of Community Homecare Research at the College of Health Professions at Thomas Jefferson University in Philadelphia.

Novel approaches to facilitating caregiving are being explored, such as teleconferencing to allow caregivers to speak in groups with a trained expert and caregiving information accessible by computer. REACH also has been fine-tuning more "old-fashioned" ways caregivers can reduce stress such as improving communication. Overall, though, REACH recommends caregivers do the best they can to make life as comfortable not just for their loved ones but for *themselves,* too.

Jealousy. As the caregiver begins to feel increasingly more isolated, feelings of jealousy may arise. The caregiver may feel specific jealousies toward family members or friends for being "free" but also a more global jealousy toward the unshackled human populace in general. Caregivers may even come to be jealous of the very person receiving their care.

Depression. The combined emotional weight of frustration, anger, loneliness, and guilt can produce, not surprisingly, depression—a condition that differs from sadness in certain key ways. While sadness usually is in response to a particular incident and has an end, depression comes from a pervasive pessimism that the future is without hope and can be dangerously self-perpetuating. Depression can lead to chronic fatigue, which in turn can worsen the depression, highlighting the importance of stopping depression *before* it has set in.

> *Depression can lead to chronic fatigue, which in turn can worsen the depression, highlighting the importance of stopping depression before it has set in.*

Grief. Grief is the price we pay for having loved someone, and it can be especially painful in the context of Alzheimer's because people with this illness can seem to die a little bit every day, Dr. Brandt says. When the end does come, it can be especially difficult for bringing on conflicting feelings of mourning combined with a sense of relief.

IF ALL ELSE FAILS . . .

If you find your caregiving responsibilities are beginning to overwhelm you and family members or friends aren't available to help, do *not* assume you're at the end of your rope. Thankfully, organizations are dedicated to the very problem you face, and many have access to volunteers willing to help out for no fee. Give one of the organizations listed the appendix under "National Organizations" a call and explain your situation. Or if you're computer-savvy, check them out at their Web addresses. You're simply too important not to get the help you need, and health officials, fortunately, have realized this.

CHAPTER 6

Finding Care Outside
the Home
Knowing When, Deciding Where

℘

*Placement [in a nursing home] is not failure. It is the only
way to ensure that someone gets 24-hour care.*

—FRENA GRAY-DAVIDSON, DIRECTOR OF SELF-HELP ALZHEIMER'S
CAREGIVER'S TRAINING AND INFORMATION

Allen had learned to handle a lot since taking on his father's care.
Over a hundred cans of ravioli in the garage "in case of an emergency." Beethoven's *Moonlight Sonata* played badly on the piano every
night well past midnight. Questions repeated so often that Allen once
screamed loud enough for the neighbors to call 911. It was the day of
the "fellings" that Allen realized that perhaps the time for outside
help had come.

One Saturday as Allen napped, his father had found an ax in the
garage and managed to cut down over a dozen fruit trees he and Allen
had planted some 20 years before. "The birds," his father said, "were
starting to drive me crazy."

"'Starting'?" Allen might have responded had he not felt such a profound sense of loss. His father seemed to bid his farewell that day. No longer would Allen be able to feel he was doing the right thing by taking charge of his father's care at home.

"Letting go of a loved one's care is one of the most difficult decisions families have to make," says Juergen Bludau, M.D., C.M.D., the medical director of the Morse Geriatric Center in West Palm Beach, Florida. Even when placing a loved one in a care facility is the unquestionably right thing to do, rarely does it feel that way. Caregivers often feel they're abandoning their loved one, Dr. Bludau says, especially spouses of people with AD who may be haunted by their vow of "until death do us part."

> *Do not feel you're failing by letting go of your loved one's care. If you take the time to find a care facility that's good, you'll be succeeding by raising your loved one's care to an even higher level.*

The goal of this chapter is to put such feelings to rest. There comes a time in this disease when finding care outside the home is in the best interests of everyone concerned, and we'll help you know when that time comes. We'll also give you a look at the wide variety of care facilities now available for people with AD, many of which offer a quality of care not just equal, but in many ways superior, to what families can provide at home. "Families need to realize that good intentions don't always make for good care," Dr. Bludau says. "As this disease progresses, it can put demands on caregivers that simply can be impossible to meet."

So no, do not feel you're failing by letting go of your loved one's care. If you take the time to find a care facility that's good, you'll be *succeeding* by raising your loved one's care to an even higher level.

KNOWING WHEN

How can you know when this time to let go has come?

We wish we could say there was an easy answer to that question, but there's not. "Every case of this illness develops so differently and the tolerance levels of caregivers can vary so widely that this is a question that needs to be answered on an individual basis," Dr. Bludau says. "A situation that's tolerable for one person might be intolerable for another, so people really need to let their individual feelings be their guide."

Dr. Bludau does offer some observations that can help bring this foggy issue into better focus, however. "Caregivers need to realize that if a situation is becoming highly stressful for them, it's also becoming highly stressful for their loved one. Caregivers often feel torn between doing what's best for their loved one and doing what's best for themselves, but really there's very little difference between the two."

Dr. Bludau mentions another point caregivers need to keep in mind: People in the middle and later stages of AD often reach a point where they need attention virtually 24 hours a day. In a nursing home or other long-term facility, this attention is provided by *three* different people working in *three* different 8-hour shifts. "Caregivers mustn't feel guilty," Dr. Bludau says, "for not being able to perform what in essence would need to be a superhuman task."

That said, here are two basic questions that shed some valuable light on the difficult issue of when to seek outside care. An affirmative answer to either should alert you that the time to make other arrangements has come.

1. Is the well-being of your loved one beginning to suffer because of difficulty you're having in providing his or her care?

2. Is your own well-being beginning to suffer because of difficulty you're having in providing this care?

Why Sooner Is Better

If your answers to these questions have you thinking that yes, perhaps the time for a care facility has come, it's important not to procrastinate. "The problems of trying to locate a good home quickly are enormous," warn Nancy Mace, M.A., and Peter Rabins, M.D., in their caregiver's guide, *The 36-Hour Day*.[1] Even if your loved one seems to be doing fine and the need for a care facility seems a long way off, the sooner you begin your search, the more satisfied you're going to be. Yes, you could wait for a crisis to occur (as many caregivers do, unfortunately), but this is not a smart way to go. As we'll be seeing in a moment, finding a really good facility can take time. Most experts recommend beginning the search as soon after diagnosis as possible, in fact, and for the following reasons.

To get the best quality. Many good and even great facilities are now available, but some "clunkers" are still out there that may take some time to weed out. You also want to make the best match possible between what you would like and what you can afford, which also can take time. If the facility you choose is a good one, it will probably have a waiting list, so you should take this likelihood into account as well. Remember, though, that finding a facility you like doesn't mean you have to use it. Usually a place can be reserved with a deposit, which will assure immediate availability or a short wait, at worst, when your time of need arrives.

> *People with AD usually have an easier time making the transition to long-term care earlier rather than later in their disease.*

To explore best sources of payment. Not only can the cost of good long-term care be considerable—between $40,000 and $70,000 a year in most areas—but the laws governing payment for this care can be complicated and vary widely from state to state. Depending on your family's or loved one's existing resources, assistance from Medicare or Medicaid may be available, but it can be a long and tedious process to find out. The bottom line, therefore, is that you improve your chances of getting insurance organizations to pay by contacting them as soon as possible.

To ease the trauma. Facilities and finances aside, another reason to get an early start at finding long-term care is that people with AD usually have an easier time making the transition when the change is made earlier rather than later in their disease. Not only are they better able to understand the reasons for the change, they're usually more capable of adapting to the surroundings of the new environment once they get there. Some adjustment trauma might still occur, causing a worsening of symptoms temporarily, but this condition usually passes in a matter of a few weeks.

To let your loved one be involved. Finally, this is a decision that your loved one is going to have to live with most of all, so it's only fair that he or she should have as much a say in the matter as possible. Alzheimer's is an illness that's progressive, remember, so the sooner you ask for such involvement, the more meaningful it's apt to be. If feasible, invite your loved to shop around for places with you, in fact, because it can be the best way to minimize the aforementioned adjustment trauma.

DECIDING WHERE

At one time, deciding on a long-term care facility for a loved one was relatively easy—although not necessarily comfortable—because the options were limited. There were nursing homes, and that was essentially it. But the increasing prevalence of AD and other age-related disabilities has altered the scene immensely. Options now range from high-tech intensive care units for people with severe disabilities to facilities resembling country clubs for the more mobile and alert.

This variety in itself highlights the importance of searching for a facility early—and searching well. "More important than the particular type of facility is the quality of the care the facility offers," says Jonathan M. Evans, M.D., a geriatrics and community internal medicine expert at the Mayo Clinic in Rochester, Minnesota. As the Alzheimer's Association reminds us, "The earlier you explore care arrangements, the more likely you are

> *Options now range from high-tech intensive care units for people with severe disabilities to facilities resembling country clubs for the more mobile and alert.*

to find a facility whose philosophy, environment, location, and price will meet your needs."

We'll give you some specific advice on what to look for in a facility in a moment, but first here's a quick rundown of the types of facilities available, along with the basic services you can expect each to provide. Facilities are discussed in the order of the degree of impairment they're intended to serve.

Retirement Housing

These facilities are for people who, for whatever reason, no longer want the responsibility of managing an entire house. Some facilities offer meal plans, housekeeping services, transportation to shopping areas, access to a health care center, and a wide range of recreational opportunities, but they generally do not provide anything in the way of specialized care for people with mental or physical impairments.

Assisted Living Facilities

Assisted living facility (ALF) is a broadly used term that can include everything from a shared apartment to larger complexes with residents numbering in the dozens. Intended to bridge the gap between living on one's own and living in a highly structured nursing home, the facilities usually provide a homey environment that includes communal dining, recreational programs, social activities, housekeeping services, and assistance with personal care. The facilities usually provide 24-hour security, emergency call systems, and assistance with medications, and are most suitable for people in the early to middle stages of AD. Their goal is to keep people with AD as active, functional, and independent as possible, for as long as possible, before other more intensive care may be required.

Nursing Homes

Nursing homes constitute the next rung up on the ladder of care for people with AD, and they are the oldest type of facility used for this purpose. Also called "intermediate care" or "skilled care" facilities, they're usually best for people in the middle to later stages of the illness or people who also have other medical problems. Because of their distinctly hospital-like environment, however, nursing homes generally are not recommended for people in earlier stages of AD who may do better in a less-restricted environment. For people with AD suffering from other medical conditions, on the other hand, or who may be in a particularly feeble stage of AD, a nursing home *is* the best place to be.

> *For people with AD suffering from other medical conditions or who may be in a particularly feeble stage of AD, a nursing home is the best place to be.*

Special Care Units

Often nursing homes will have a special care units (SCU) set up for the care of people with Alzheimer's disease, featuring a calm, homey environment and staffed by members specially trained in dealing with the illness. Sometimes these SCUs are "special" in name only, however, offering few advantages over the rest of the facility. If you're considering an SCU, be sure to ask the person in charge what makes it special. If the answer appears to be little more than a sign on a locked door, continue your search.

Continuum Care Retirement Communities

The concept of continuum care retirement communities (CCRCs) is conveyed in the word *continuum*. The facilities offer residents the opportunity to continue living at the same basic complex through various stages of their later years, thus eliminating the need for disruptive moves as a medical condition may grow worse. In what's known as the "retirement" section of a CCRC, for example, few services are offered, making this section appropriate for people who are fully functional or only moderately impaired. As a resident's degree of impairment may increase, however, other sections of the facility or levels of service are made available. While some CCRCs require that

High Standards of Care

Recently a private, not-for-profit agency called the Joint Commission on Accreditation of Healthcare Organizations has been formed for the purpose of improving the quality of health care facilities of many types. While accreditation by this commission is not yet mandatory, some facilities have complied to the Joint Commission's high standards voluntarily and thus should be considered good choices.

residents be relatively independent at the time of admission, others do not. The services offered by CCRCs can vary widely, as can the financial terms for acquiring them, so be prepared to ask lots of questions (see some suggestions later) of any CCRC you may consider.

Hospice Care

Hospice care is available through special hospice organizations but also many nursing homes, hospitals, and other types of heath care agencies. The purpose of a hospice service is to provide comfort and care to people in the end stages of an illness, but without the use of dramatic lifesaving measures. Hospice care is covered by Medicare, some insurance plans, and Medicaid in some states, but only if a physician makes an official determination in advance that the person is not expected to live beyond 6 months. (For more information on a hospice service in your area, check under "Hospices" in the classified section of the phone book.)

KNOWING THE GOOD FROM THE BAD

We'd like to say that every health care facility available for the long-term care of people with AD and other dementias was a haven run by compassionate professionals dedicated to treating your loved one as tenderly as they would treat their own, but unfortunately some of these facilities fall short. They may be understaffed, underfunded, and simply not capable of providing the level of care your loved one deserves.

Various organizations are making efforts to improve the quality of long-term care in the United States, but for the time being, the bulk of the responsibility still rests with people like you—the consumers who need to judge the adequacy of a care facility on their own. You should do some preliminary investigation before signing on any dotted lines to feel confident that quality care will be provided, for not just your loved one's physical needs but his or her emotional, social, and spiritual ones as well, says Dr. Evans. Here are some tips from Dr. Evans, the Alzheimer's Association, and some other leading AD experts on how to find a facility you can feel confident will be managing your loved one in a caring and competent manner:

> Various organizations are making efforts to improve the quality of long-term care in the United States, but for the time being, the bulk of the responsibility still rests with people like you—the consumers who need to judge the adequacy of a care facility on their own.

- Begin your search as early as possible. A lot of time and consideration should go into the decision process, and you don't want to be caught short and have to make it in a rush. Don't be afraid to say no to those facilities that don't meet your approval. This is a decision that you as well as your loved one are going to have to live with, possibly for quite some time.

- Visit the facility several times and at different times of the day to get a feel for the atmosphere and how things are being done. Do residents seem to be getting personal attention, or are they spending most of their time in front of TVs in their wheelchairs? Are they being treated with respect by staff members? Take along another family member or friend with whom your observations can be shared.

Don't Forget Adult Day Care

While the term *day care* may be offensive to some because of its "childish" connotation, the services provided by these facilities can be invaluable. "I don't know what I'd so without it," says one caregiver we talked to. "And my husband adores going. Even if he's cranky, he always comes home in a better mood."

Adult day care centers can help bridge the gap between full-time care at home and full-time care at a long-term facility, providing caregivers breaks whenever they're needed most. Hours usually are very flexible, allowing caregivers to drop their loved ones off for just a few hours or the entire day. In addition to providing meals and a wide variety of recreational activities supervised by trained professionals, some centers also dispense medications, provide transporta-

- Talk with family members of other residents to get their views on the quality of care their loved ones have been receiving. Have they had complaints, and if so, has the staff been responsive at making amends?

- Use your nose, being on the lookout for smells of urine, especially, which may indicate poor attention to care in other areas as well.

- Check out the dining facilities and ask to see a week's menu. Notice, too, how residents are being assisted if they need help. Are they being force-fed or given time to eat at their own pace?

- Peruse as much of the facility as possible. A good one will be warm and cheerily decorated on the inside and offer ample opportunity for activities outside such as walking, gardening, and playing with pets. If your loved one has been used to taking walks, the provisions for this activity will be especially importion, and assist with personal tasks such as eating and bathing. Most centers are open 5 or 6 days a week during normal business hours and cost in about $50 a day. This cost may qualify as an itemized deduction for medical expenses, however, or could be covered by another provision known as the Household and Dependent Care Credit, explained later. Some centers also adjust fees according to a sliding scale for those in need, and discounts usually are available for people who attend daily.

For more information on a center near you, check with your local hospital or your loved one's doctor. The National Council on Aging also keeps information on an extensive list of centers (phone: [202] 479-1200), as does Eldercare Locator ([800] 677-1116) and your state's department on aging.

---

tant. Best of all is a circular path that goes through natural surroundings yet is well secured.

- Request to see the facility's most recent *facility inspection report*, an evaluation that should be done regularly by a state inspection agency. You also can contact your local ombudsman office, a federally run agency that records and oversees complaints about long-term health care facilities in every state.

- Ask for a description of the facility's basic philosophy of care. Are provisions made for adapting to each resident's individual needs, or is the approach more "cookie-cutter" style in which one basic plan is intended to accommodate all?

- Ask to see the facility's activities schedule. It should include a good variety, including music, art, socialization activities, exercise opportunities, and crafts.

- Find out whether activities are offered on a group as well as an individual basis. A mix is best, because group activities can help residents maintain skills important for communication with others.

- Talk with members of the staff to see how certain specific situations might be handled. Mention any particularly peculiar behaviors your loved one may have to see how the staff would respond. If you don't like what you hear, you may need to continue your search.

For more information on how to choose a reliable health care facility, call the Alzheimer's Association ([800] 272-3900) and request the following publications free of charge:

Respite Care: How to Find What's Right for You

Residential Care: A Guide for Choosing a New Home

Services You May Need Fact Sheet

Making the Visits Less Vexing

Sherry Bell had cared for her mother at home for many years, and although she had experienced difficulties, never had she felt as uneasy as when she visited her mother at the nursing home. "Knowing how to visit did not come naturally," Sherry says of the awkwardness she felt. Not wanting her relationship with her mother to end, she decided to do whatever she could to make her visits both pleasant and meaningful; before she knew it, Sherry had enough insight for a book. The book, *Visiting Mom, an Unexpected Gift: A Guide for Visiting Elders with Alzheimer's*, is a warehouse of helpful tips, some of which are listed here:

- When visiting, expect to be visiting not just your loved one but perhaps also a host of roommates, friends, and even health care attendants.

- Forget using conventional greetings that harmlessly ask such questions as "Hi, how are you," or "So, how's it going?" These questions are not likely to be met with positive answers or any

answers at all. It's better to keep greetings positive and state-
ments rather than questions, Bell says, such as, "Good to see
you again," or "Hi! You're looking well today."

- Beware of asking your loved one too many questions. You may
  tend to want to know a lot of details on the care your loved one
  is receiving, but it puts an undue pressure on the resident to
  expect him or her to be able to verbalize the answers. Instead,
  direct your questions at staff members.

- Go equipped with tangible and intangible "props" to keep the
  conversation moving and to help your loved one feel more at
  home in the new surroundings, such as old family photos, me-
  mentos, and stories that recall fond memories.

- Spend time doing some kind of activity or craft your loved one
  may still be capable of, or go for a walk or listen to the person's
  favorite music. "Tony Bennett has changed our lives," Bell says
  of a musical pastime she and her mother
  particularly enjoy together.

> *Spend time doing some kind of activity or craft your loved one may still be capable of, or go for a walk or listen to the person's favorite music.*

- Come with a special bag of treats, such as
  fresh fruit, flowers, a favorite dessert, or
  special soap. Check with the facility first,
  if need be, to make sure your loved one
  isn't following special dietary guidelines
  that edible treats might overstep.

- Spend time with grooming activities, such
  as combing hair or doing nails.

- Expect to be flexible, because moods can vary widely from visit
  to visit. Also be ready for capabilities and demeanor to decline
  gradually due to the progressive nature of this disease.

- Be ready to answer the question of "When am I going home?"
  by explaining that the facility *is* your loved one's home, stressing all its positive features such as the enjoyable activities, nutritious food, and good friends.

- Do your best to see and express the humor in things, an aid to making you both feel more at ease.

- Conclude visits by reassuring your loved one you'll be returning soon, and do it while you're still seated to make the announcement seem less imminent and ominous.[2]

FINANCIAL AFFAIRS

As challenging as Alzheimer's disease can be emotionally and physically, it can impose considerable financial burdens as well. The out-of-pocket cost of caring for someone with AD at home averages over $12,000 a year, the Alzheimer's Association reports, while full-time residential care can range between $40,000 and $70,000 depending on the facility. Thankfully, various insurance programs, medical benefits, and other financial resources often can help cover some of these costs, but you may need some financial savvy to obtain them.

> *Various insurance programs, medical benefits, and other financial resources often can help cover some of these costs, but you may need some financial savvy to obtain them.*

We'll summarize as best we can the resources available, but it can be wise to consult with a financial adviser to be sure you'll be getting all the assistance due to you by law. Check with your local chapter of the Alzheimer's Association if you're uncertain about how to contact a financial adviser or if you have any other questions regarding legal or financial issues. The person you talk to will be able to give you a referral list of qualified professionals including financial planners, accountants, and attorneys specializing in issues encountered by the elderly. In the meantime, here are some general tips on how to manage what can be some fairly complicated legal and financial matters relating to this disease:

Start early. As a caregiver, you may be responsible for a wide range of financial duties, including paying bills, arranging for benefit claims, making investment decisions, and preparing tax returns, so the sooner

The Eden Alternative: Children, a Garden, and a Flock of Laying Hens

As an example of the new heights being achieved by long-term care facilities these days, consider a facility known as the Eden Alternative at the Chase Memorial Nursing Home in New Berlin, New York. The "core concept" of the facility, according to its medical director, William Thomas, M.D., is that nursing homes should be "habitats for human beings rather than institutions for the frail and elderly."[3] True to that goal, residents are encouraged to interact with children who attend a day care center, an after-school program, and a summer camp located on the "campus," as it's called. Campus members live in small, family-style groups made up of people whose cognitive abilities are similar to encourage social interaction, and participation in day-to-day activities such as meal preparation, dressing, and personal grooming are encouraged as much as possible. A wide variety of activities are offered indoors, while residents are invited outdoors to work in a large vegetable and flower garden, take walks, and enjoy the company of animals including dogs, cats, rabbits, and even a flock of egg-producing hens. "The Eden Alternative seeks to eliminate the three plagues of long-term institutions: loneliness, helplessness and boredom," Dr. Thomas says.

you can begin investigating these matters, the better. Remember to get professional help if you need it.

Involve your loved one. Another reason to get an early start is to maximize the level of input you'll be able to get from your loved one before communication regarding such affairs might become more difficult. Find out what the person with AD would like done with his or her financial resources.

Involve other family members. Get other relatives' ideas on how your loved one's finances and long-term care should be managed. If considerable costs are to be accrued, be sure to find out their willingness to contribute.

Take inventory. This means doing a thorough review of all your loved one's relevant legal and financial documents including wills, powers of attorney (see the sidebar "Important Legal Concerns"), insurance policies, stock and bond certificates, bank and brokerage account information, pension and other retirement benefit summaries, Social Security information, deeds or mortgage papers, possible inheritance due in the future, and any monthly or outstanding bills. If you use a financial planner, all this information will be required.

> *A*nother reason to get an early start is to maximize the level of input you'll be able to get from your loved one before communication regarding such affairs might become more difficult.

Review your own financial affairs. This step can help you determine the type and extent of long-term care for your loved one you'll be able to afford. Take note of all your savings, investments, and insurance. If your loved one is financially dependent on you, you may be able to qualify for medical expense deductions and dependent care credits on your tax return.

What to Expect from Insurance

What help might you expect from your health insurance company in paying for the costs of caring for someone with AD?

Not enough, unfortunately, which has more than a few health experts advocating change. Until changes are made, however, the bulk of the financial burden of caring for people with AD and many other chronic conditions must be borne by them and their families. Most health insurance policies cover the costs of *acute* illnesses, not chronic ones, and while the benefits of these policies may include hospitalization, physician fees, and outpatient tests, these usually make up only a small portion of the care people with AD need.

This reality doesn't mean that financial assistance for AD care isn't available, however, especially for people in financial need. Here's quick rundown of the types of assistance caregivers and their families may be able to access.

Medicare

Thanks to a landmark decision made by the Bush administration in March of 2002, Medicare (the federal health insurance program for Americans 65 and older and also people younger than 65 who have been on Social Security disability for at least 24 months) must now include treatment for Alzheimer's disease. Such treatment includes mental health services, physical therapy and occupational therapy, medications, hospice care, and care provided at home, thus greatly relieving financial burdens imposed on caregivers and their families. Before this ruling, reimbursement for many AD treatments had been denied based on the assumption that such treatments were futile—a notion that recent studies have found ample reason to refute. Also influential in the policy shift have been recent improvements in the ability of doctors to diagnose AD in its early stages, thus improving the likelihood of treatments achieving meaningful effects. For more information on the benefits provided by Medicare, call (800) 638-6833 or check its Web site at www.medicare.gov.

Medicaid

Medicaid is funded jointly by the federal and state governments and will pay for medical care for people with very low incomes, including long-term care for people who have depleted their resources. Most Medicaid funds go toward providing care in nursing homes, but some states have begun to pay for other types of long-term care as well. Not all long-term care facilities accept payment from Medicaid, however, so choices can be limited. To learn more about Medicaid, contact your

Important Legal Concerns

Certain legal issues can get quite messy if they're not taken care of early in the course of Alzheimer's disease, so it's best to get them taken care of as soon as possible for the peace of mind of everyone concerned. First, it will be necessary for you to have a lawyer create what's called a *durable power of attorney*, a legal document that empowers a specified person to make decisions regarding legal and financial issues on behalf of the person with AD after he or she is no longer able to do. The sooner this step is done the better, because it requires the person with AD to be sufficiently competent to give a signed consent.

Also to be discussed and established as soon as possible is a *living will*, a document that specifies what medical treatments or life sup-

state or county human services or social services department in the blue pages of your phone book.

Long-Term Care Insurance

This type of insurance can be a godsend in that it usually will cover most of the expenses that the long-term care of people with AD can incur. It also can be prohibitively expensive, however, and needs to be purchased before a diagnosis of AD is made. Because programs offered by different companies can vary widely, moreover, the Alzheimer's Association recommends that prospective buyers ask the following questions to be sure they're getting what they want:

- Is Alzheimer's disease covered? (Do not assume that it is unless clearly specified.)

- How impaired does the person with AD have to be before benefits can be collected? (Policies usually are very specific about this point but also can be a quite stingy.)

port procedures the person with AD might wish—or not wish—to have employed as the end of the illness draws near.

Last, while the person with Alzheimer's is still capable, discuss what he or she would like done with assets. A *living trust,* whereby a person's assets are put into a fund managed by someone of the person's choice, often works well.

As you can see, all of these matters require a certain degree of mental competence, so the sooner you can get them taken care of, the less difficulty you're likely to have. Keep in mind, too, that laws governing the elderly's legal concerns can vary so widely and are changing so rapidly that an attorney specializing in elder care in general—and Alzheimer's disease in particular—probably will be able to serve you best. Check with the Alzheimer's Association in your area for the names of good candidates.

- Exactly what types of care does the policy cover?

- How large will the reimbursements be, and will they be adjusted annually for inflation?

- How long will reimbursements continue to be paid?

- Will reimbursements be made immediately upon diagnosis, or must some time elapse?

- Will any tax need to be paid on the reimbursements received?

Life Insurance

Life insurance can be a valuable source of payment for long-term care, the Alzheimer's Association says. "You may be able to borrow from a policy's cash value, or the person with AD may be able to receive a portion of the policy's face value as a loan," experts there explain.[4] Called a *viatical loan,* it can be paid off at the time of death. Some life insurance policies also feature a *waiver of premium rider,* which means the person insured does not have to pay for continued coverage if he or she becomes disabled—worth looking into, for sure.

Help from Other Sources

Fortunately, insurance policies aren't the only way to help defray the costs of caring for a loved one with AD. Funds from various governmental programs also are available to help lighten the load provided a sufficient financial need exists.

Social Security Disability Insurance (SSDI). Financial aid from this organization is available to people under the age of 65 who qualify as disabled according to the standards established by the Social Security Administration. Usually this condition requires proof that the person is unable to work at any occupation or that the person is suffering from a condition expected to result in death within 1 year. It's important to apply for SSDI as soon as possible because in addition to taking a long time to be reviewed, applications often are rejected the first time through, necessitating an appeal.

> *It's important to apply for SSDI as soon as possible because in addition to taking a long time to be reviewed, applications often are rejected the first time through, necessitating an appeal.*

Supplemental Security Income (SSI). This program makes monthly payments available to people with limited incomes who are 65 or older or who are disabled or blind. As with SSDI, applications can take a long time to be approved, so people with AD are encouraged to begin the application as soon after diagnosis as possible. For more information on both SSDI and SSI, you can call the Social Security Administration at (800) 772-1213 or check its Web site at www.ssa.gov.

Veteran's Benefits. Although this resource has been declining in recent years, some benefits for people with AD and other chronic health problems may still be available. To explore this option, you may contact the Department of Veteran's Affairs at (800) 733-8387.

Other Public Programs. Alzheimer's disease has become such a widespread problem that many communities have managed to organize facilities offering short-term as well as long-term care by using state funds. Check with your local chapter of the Alzheimer's Association or the Department (or Council) on Aging in your state to find what's available in your area. You also can get information on these services by calling the Eldercare Locator Service at (800) 677-1116.

Tax Benefits. Yes, even the Internal Revenue Service has developed a place in its heart for caregivers of people with AD. If you're still employed and can qualify the person with AD as a dependent, you may be able to use the Household and Dependent Care Credit to deduct expenses for care directly from the amount of tax you otherwise would owe.

The Family Medical Leave Act. This provision doesn't provide money but rather time. It requires that companies of 50 or more people must grant up to 12 weeks of unpaid leave a year to any employee needing to care for a parent, spouse, or child suffering from a serious health problem, AD included. The 12 weeks can be taken all at once or in segments, and in addition to continuing to provide all health benefits during this time, the employer must guarantee a position of equal status and pay when the leave has expired. Eligibility requires having worked at the company for at least 12 months (or 1,250 hours) and obtaining medical certification of the illness requiring care.

HAPPY ENDINGS

But you'd simply never be able to live with yourself if you relinquished the care of your loved one? Allen (mentioned before) had the same fears, but he learned they were ungrounded. Allen had chosen a facility near enough to home that he could visit his dad several times a week, and from what Allen could see, his father appeared surprisingly happy—happier, in fact, than he had been at home. "I think Dad knew he was becoming a burden, and it was upsetting him in ways that added to his agitation. I think he may even have been as relieved as I was once we got him settled in his new situtation. He made friends and even rediscovered some old hobbies. I have a painting he did hanging in my office, and not just because I like it, but because it helps remind me I did the right thing."

What Allen's story shows is that "right" decisions rarely feel right at the time we need to make them. Time is needed to verify the wisdom of our most difficult choices, so we need to be patient. Keep in mind, too, that the expression of love needn't be dependent on locale. The quality of the time you have left with your loved one will depend on what you choose to make it. Many people find they're able to be even more giving of affection, in fact, when not stressed with having to care for their loved ones on a daily basis.

As for feeling guilty, "it's a useless emotion," says Dr. Brandt. "Give what you can and don't worry about what you can't." Just as the young eventually need to leave the nest, so, too, may the old.

CHAPTER 7

The Anti-Alzheimer's Lifestyle

❦

We need to take care of our bodies and our basic health
when we're younger in order to help lower our risk
for Alzheimer's disease later in life.

—*STEVE SEINER, M.D., INSTRUCTOR OF PSYCHIATRY*
AT HARVARD MEDICAL SCHOOL

As doctors work to treat Alzheimer's disease, caregivers struggle to manage it, and the health care system worries about how to afford it, the question looms ever larger: Might there be ways we can prevent Alzheimer's disease in the first place? It's a question we certainly deserve to ask as we take our walks, steam our broccoli, and read our *Prevention* magazines in hopes of living longer. If preserving our bodies is only going to earn us the time it takes to lose our minds, after all, what's the point?

Relax, and keep steaming the broccoli. Scientists are finding that by preserving our bodies, we *are* helping preserve our minds. "There's no question that we can reduce our risks of this disease by taking care of ourselves in some very fundamental ways," says Paul Raia, Ph.D., the director of patient care for the Alzheimer's Association in Cambridge, Massachusetts. "What we're finding is that what's good for the heart also tends to be good for the brain, so by controlling things such as blood pressure, cholesterol levels, and body weight, people also are helping to control their risks for Alzheimer's disease."

But it also appears we can enlist our brains themselves to work in their own defense against the illness, with surprising results. Studies have begun to show that by engaging in intellectually stimulating activities such as reading, writing, playing a musical instrument, doing puzzles, or playing chess, we may be able to build enough brain power in reserve to help us escape the effects of AD even if it should develop.

> Studies have begun to show that by engaging in intellectually stimulating activities such as reading, writing, playing a musical instrument, doing puzzles, or playing chess, we may be able to build enough brain power in reserve to help us escape the effects of AD even if it should develop.

"All in all, it's an encouraging picture that seems to be emerging," says Dr. Raia concerning the control we may have over this seemingly uncontrollable disease. "The more we learn about Alzheimer's, in fact, the more we're finding that by reducing our risks, we may be able to reduce our risks for other serious health problems as well."

In this chapter we'll see how. We'll start by examining the findings of a remarkable study that's been investigating how certain healthy habits have been reducing risks for Alzheimer's disease within a uniquely isolated population of nuns. Then we'll see how these findings coincide encouragingly with discoveries from other studies being done worldwide. Along the way, we'll see how we can incorporate the results of these studies into our own lives.

HEALTHY HABITS: LESSONS LEARNED FROM THE NUN STUDY

"Outside of a laboratory, it would be hard to find as pure an environment for research." That statement is how David Snowdon, Ph.D., a professor of neurology at the University of Kentucky Medical Center, describes the context of a study he's been directing for the past 16 years that stands to be among the most important of its kind in helping unlock AD's long-held secrets.[1] Since 1986, Dr. Snowdon has been monitoring the health and habits of 678 Catholic sisters between the ages of 75 and 106 whose restricted lifestyles have made them near-perfect subjects for revealing what may be the greatest risk factors for developing this disease. The women have had the same basic routines, the same access to health care, and even similar diets for decades, allowing Dr. Snowdon to weed out many of the variables that so often can confuse population studies of this type.

Making the study even more unique, Dr. Snowdon has been permitted to do autopsies of the women's brains upon death, thus allowing him to know without a doubt their Alzheimer's status. Armed with this critical information, the remaining challenge for Dr. Snowdon and his staff has been to determine in each woman's case what might have been unique about her life to encourage—or discourage—AD onset. Especially illuminating, Dr. Snowdon reports, have been his studies of sisters in pairs. "The more closely two sisters' lives overlap and yet have different outcomes, the more readily we've been able to identify factors that may have led to their different fates," he explains.[2]

What sort of "factors" has Dr. Snowdon been finding? Factors well within our power to control, as the following sections explain.

The Importance of Mental Exercise: Building Brain Power in Reserve

Researchers have suspected for some time that mental activity might help protect against the effects of AD, but not until the Nun Study would such shocking proof emerge. Snowdon and his team found that some of the women who had led intellectually stimulating lives had been able to remain highly functional right up until their time of death even though their autopsies showed brain damage from AD that was shockingly severe. Other sisters who had led less intellectually active lives, by contrast, were found to be highly dysfunctional at the time of death despite autopsies showing their damage from AD to be relatively mild.

"The results stunned us," Dr. Snowdon admits, but after some reflection, he and his team had theorized an answer: The mentally active women may have built up a reserve of neurological pathways that allowed their brains essentially to "work around" the damage AD had caused.[3] Whether or not mental activity can prevent Alzheimer's disease, therefore, it at least may be able to ameliorate its effects, Dr. Snowdon says.

The Importance of Physical Exercise: Improving the Brain's Fuel Supply

Sister Nicolette, one of the most robust sisters in Dr. Snowdon's study and still alert at age 91, attributed her health to walking 2 miles every day, a routine she had started at the age of 70. Her agile frame aside, what might Sister Nicolette's routine have been doing for her brain? "Exercise improves blood flow," Dr. Snowdon explains, "bringing the brain the oxygen and nutrients it needs to function well. It also reduces stress hormones and increases chemicals that nourish brain cells, which can help ward off depression and some kinds of damage to brain tissue." Exercise

> *Exercise also can help prevent strokes, diabetes, high blood pressure, and high cholesterol—all of which can elevate AD risks.*

also can help prevent strokes, diabetes, high blood pressure, and high cholesterol—all of which can elevate AD risks. Small wonder, then, that Dr. Snowdon should have such a quick and easy answer to the question he's so often asked about the single most important thing we should do as we age. "Walk" is his one-word reply.[4]

New Nutritional Links

While other research has pointed to the importance of antioxidant vitamins such as vitamins E and C in safeguarding the brain, Dr. Snowdon's study has found that two other nutrients also may be important: lycopene and folate (also known as folic acid). Lycopene, which Dr. Snowdon has found to be associated with longevity more than any other nutrient tested in his study, is a powerful antioxidant with a reddish color. Folate, on the other hand, appears to protect the brain directly by joining forces with another B vitamin (B_{12}) to guard brain cells from the toxic effects of a substance known as homocysteine. Best folate sources are leafy green vegetables, dried beans, citrus fruits, liver, and nuts, while lycopene is best gotten from cooked tomato products eaten along with some dietary fat, Dr. Snowdon says—good news for lovers of pizza and spaghetti, he notes.

Double Trouble from Depression

Might depression increase risks of Alzheimer's disease? Dr. Snowdon is beginning to think so. In addition to evidence from his own study, he cites research showing that a history of depression can increase risks of developing AD by nearly twofold. Whether chronic depression might stress brain cells in unusual ways, scientists aren't sure, but they have found that chronic depression can cause a shrinkage of the hippocampus (the memory center) of the brain in a manner suspiciously similar to what's seen in people with AD. As a result, depression may work in tandem with Alzheimer's disease, Dr. Snowdon says, to make the symptoms of AD even worse.[5]

Reasons to Keep Your Spirits High

If depression can increase risks of AD, might cheeriness have just the opposite effect? Dr. Snowdon is still collecting data to answer that question, but he has found that a positive outlook can help defend against disease in general. After studying autobiographies that 178 of the sisters in his study had written back in their 20s, his team was able to find a definite connection between "positive emotional content" and the longest life spans. Astonished by the results, Snowdon and his crew reexamined their data from a number of angles but each time came up with the same results. "From the low to the high end of the scale, positive emotions had accounted for a survival difference of 6.9 years," Dr. Snowdon says. When the researchers studied their figures in yet another way, they found that women who had told of the greatest sorrows were at twice the risk for death at all ages compared to those who had told of the greatest joys.[6]

BEST WAYS TO KEEP AD AT BAY

While the Nun Study has been among the most publicized research projects looking into how Alzheimer's disease might be associated with lifestyle, by no means has it been the only one. Researchers worldwide have been investigating AD for its possible lifestyle links since the early 1990s, and they've been finding some intriguing connections. What we eat, how we exercise, even how we handle stress and manage our emotions—all can affect the health of our brains in subtle but important ways and may influence our chances of developing Alzheimer's disease as a result. As explained by William Li, M.D., a clinical instructor of medicine at Harvard Medical School and the president and medical director of the Angiogenesis Foundation in Cambridge, Massachusetts: "We're beginning to see Alzheimer's as a disease not just with a single cause but rather as an illness much like cancer that develops slowly due to many causes involving a series of breakdowns within several of the body's different systems. It can only make sense, therefore, to keep each of these systems functioning as well as possible to reduce the likelihood of Alzheimer's."

> When the researchers studied their figures in yet another way, they found that women who had told of the greatest sorrows were at twice the risk for death at all ages compared to those who had told of the greatest joys.

Like a chain made of many links, in other words, our defense against Alzheimer's disease may only be as strong as the weakest link.

To avoid the illness, therefore, research suggests we would do best to employ the kind of "full-body" approach outlined here.

Use Your Brain, Don't Lose It

"Like push-ups for the brain," says neuropsychologist Glenn Hammel, Ph.D., of the brain-building powers of mental stimulation. Whether it's by reading a good book, writing a thoughtful letter, playing a game of chess, or even just trying to figure out "Heart and Soul" on the piano, we expand our web of neuronal connections each time we push our brains a little further beyond their current realm, Dr. Hammel says. By establishing these connections, moreover, we create a supply in reserve that some studies suggest may help us avoid noticeable effects from brain damage such as the kind caused by Alzheimer's disease. "The theory is that cognitive reserve may act as a cushion against intellectual impairment," says Margaret Gatz, Ph.D., a professor of psychology at the University of Southern California at Los Angeles who has found evidence of this phenomenon by studying education levels in twins.[7]

Perhaps the most dramatic evidence for the "use it or lose it" theory comes from a study reported in the *Proceedings of the National Academy of Sciences* that looked at how people had spent their leisure time during their early adulthood and middle age. Even after controlling for education levels and profession, the researchers found that people whose favorite leisure-time activities had been mentally challenging ones (for example, reading, playing chess or a musical instrument, writing, or doing puzzles) proved to be two and a half times less likely to develop AD later in life (after the age of 70) than people who had preferred more intellectually passive activities, such as talking on the phone, listening to music, or watching TV.[8]

> *Researchers found that people whose favorite leisure-time activities had been mentally challenging ones (for example, reading, playing chess or a musical instrument, writing, or doing puzzles) proved to be two and a half times less likely to develop AD.*

"The brain is an organ just like every other organ in the body and it ages in regard to how it's used," remarked the study's lead author, Robert P. Friedland, M.D., a professor of neurology at Case Western Reserve University School of Medicine regarding the results. "Just as physical activity strengthens the heart, muscles, and bones against disease, intellectual activity strengthens the brain."[9] Dr. Hammel agrees. "We should think of our brains as batteries in reverse," he says, "in that they get stronger rather than weaker with use."

The take-home advice? Use your brain whenever you can. Read more; watch TV less. Write letters instead of buying cards. Take up a musical instrument. Sign up for a night course. Try using your brain instead of a pocket calculator when working with numbers or a dictionary instead of spell-check when writing on a computer. It's amazing how modern technology has made an industry out of doing some of our most basic brainwork for us.

Nourish Your Brain with Exercise

After a few chapters of *War and Peace*, you might want to take a brisk walk to help this saga sink in. As many of our greatest thinkers throughout history knew and scientists are just now beginning to understand, it seems our brains like a good bout of exercise as much as our bodies do. Consider, for example, that Beethoven wrote some of his most brilliant music in his head while taking day-long walks around Vienna, and many of Einstein's thoughts allegedly would come to him "afoot."

As many of our greatest thinkers throughout history knew and scientists are just now beginning to understand, it seems our brains like a good bout of exercise as much as our bodies do.

How might physical exercise benefit the brain? By keeping it well nourished with a robust blood flow for one thing, as noted by Dr. Snowdon, but some other important mechanisms also may be involved. In a study reported in the *Proceedings of the National Academy of Sciences*, for example, researchers have found that mice en-

It's Not Called the "Boob Tube" for Nothing

Picture the following scenario: Struggling to solve a problem, a neuron in your brain reaches outward with tentacle-like projections in hopes of making a connection that will help you arrive at a solution. If the right connection is made, not only is the problem solved, but the connection joins your lifelong collection of millions of others like it and becomes the stuff of which your basic "brain power" is made. But not only is your brain now smarter for this additional connection, it's also more durable. With one more highway added to its neurological road map, your brain is now more capable of bypassing any roadblocks—such as the plaques and tangles of Alzheimer's disease—that may come its way.

There's just one problem. We can't build these new connections in our brains by watching reruns of *Happy Days.* We need to challenge our gray matter to form these new neuronal pathways, and as funny as The Fonz may be, he's not a brain builder. TV in general appears to be something of a wasteland for our intellects, in fact, as suggested by a study reported in the *Proceedings of the National Academy of Sciences.* The purpose of the study was to determine the effects of leisure-time activities during early adulthood and middle age on risks for developing Alzheimer's disease later in life, the results of which might want to make you lose your TV for good. The favorite activity reported by virtually every one of the 193 people in the 555-person survey who had developed Alzheimer's disease was . . . yes, the "tube." People in the survey who had reported being interested in more mentally demanding activities, on the other hand, had reduced their risks of developing AD by over 50 percent.[10]

couraged to "work out" by running on exercise wheels not only added new brain cells to the memory centers of their brains but also benefited from a boost in electrical activity called *long-term potentiation* (LTP), believed to be the neurological "voltage" needed to help memories actually form. Better yet, the exercised mice performed significantly better than nonexercised mice in learning to escape from a maze, suggesting their neurological improvements had not been just "in their heads."[11]

Extrapolating these results to humans, "Physical activity may be one way to maintain and or even improve cognitive function as we age," remarked officials from the National Institute on Aging and National Institutes of Health on the study's results. "We may even be able to stimulate brain repair mechanisms by exercising," these experts say—good news, indeed, given the loss of brain cells AD is known to cause.[12]

Might there be some real-world evidence of the kind of protection these scientists are talking about? In the study mentioned earlier by Dr. Friedland, physical activity was found to be protective against AD in the same way that mental activity had. "We found that people with higher levels of activity were about three and a half times less likely to get Alzheimer's disease than those with lower levels," Dr. Friedland says.[13]

> *A*pproximately 30 minutes a day of moderate-intensity activity such as walking, cycling, participating in recreational sports, or even just doing chores around the house are all we need to shoot for.

As for the amount of exercise needed to help preserve our intellects, there's even better news. Most major health organizations, including the American College of Sports Medicine, the National Institutes of Health, the American Heart Association, and the Office of the Surgeon General, now agree that approximately 30 minutes a day of moderate-intensity activity such as walking, cycling, participating in recreational sports, or even just doing chores around the house are all we need to shoot for. More important than intensity, researchers are finding, is consistency. As Dr. Snowdon says, "The key point is to find some sort of sport or activity that you truly enjoy, so that you will do it regularly—at least 4 days a week for the rest of your life. This not only protects your heart and bones; it protects your brain."[14]

Protect Your Brain from Injury

But even a Ph.D. in nuclear physics and the ability to run a marathon can't protect against what researchers say is the third leading cause of Alzheimer's disease, behind only age and family history: a history of blows to the head. Researchers have suspected for some time that a history of head traumas can lead to the development of AD—especially any injury resulting in a loss of consciousness lasting 15 minutes or more—but not until a study by scientists from the University of Pennsylvania School of Medicine did they have such dramatic proof. Using anesthetized pigs, the researchers duplicated conditions that characterize what happens to the human brain during many car accidents—a very rapid acceleration followed by an equally rapid deceleration without actual head impact. Studying the pigs afterward, the researchers found that despite the brain's built-in elasticity and internal cushioning devices, these forces had been enough to cause the animals to suffer diffuse axonal injury (DAI) whereby nerve fibers (axons) connecting nerve cells within the brain had actually snapped.[15]

A history of head traumas can lead to the development of AD—especially any injury resulting in a loss of consciousness lasting 15 minutes or more.

Were this not injurious enough, the researchers later observed that the damaged nerve fibers started to produce a sticky substance called *A-beta*, believed to lay the foundation for the development of the Alzheimer's trademark amyloid plaques. "Our study suggests that even moderate brain injury resulting from a tremendous change-in-velocity can cause axonal damage sufficient to launch an insidiously progressive degenerative process," says Douglas H. Smith, M.D., the study's lead author and associate professor of neurosurgery at the University of Pennsylvania School of Medicine.[16]

In addition to being an important step forward for Alzheimer's research, the study highlights the importance of protecting ourselves as well as our children from head trauma, especially early in life when such injuries would have an even longer period of time to gestate into significant plaque buildup. This means diligent use of seat belts and appropriate car seats for small children in automobiles and also helmets when skating or riding bicycles, motorcycles, or scooters. (*Note:* Some researchers are concerned that a technique called "heading" employed in soccer may increase Alzheimer's risks, and while the American Academy of Pediatricians considers the danger insufficient to ban heading entirely, it does recommend that the technique be minimized until more safety studies have been done.)

> *Fruits and vegetables are our best natural sources of antioxidants, the potent disease-fighting compounds that appear to help guard brain cells against damage from free radicals—tissue-damaging molecules that scientists feel may play a critical role in the onset, as well as proliferation, of the disease.*

Feed Your Brain Lots of Fruits and Vegetables

Heralded already by the American Heart Association and American Cancer Society, a diet rich in fruits and vegetables may be an edible answer to reducing risks of Alzheimer's disease. As Dr. Snowdon says of his own efforts to improve his odds against AD, "The most important component of my health investment portfolio is eating a wide range of fresh fruits and vegetables. Promising nutrients are being discovered in plant foods that go well beyond the standard vitamins and minerals and appear to have a wide range of health-promoting effects."[17]

With respect to Alzheimer's disease, researchers are finding that diets rich in fruits and vegetables appear to exert their protective effect in several ways. Such diets can help prevent strokes, which Dr. Snowdon's study has found can increase risks for AD by over twenty-fold, but their effect also may be more direct. Fruits and vegetables are our best natural sources of antioxidants, the potent disease-fighting compounds that appear to help guard brain cells against damage from free radicals—tissue-damaging molecules that scientists feel may play a critical role in the onset, as well as proliferation, of the disease.

Which fruits and veggies help neutralize free radicals best? Listed here are those that researchers from Tufts University have found to be our best antioxidant sources. Scientists measure a food's antioxidant potential in units called *oxygen radical absorbency capacities* (ORACs), and while the USDA estimates that most of us currently take in only about 1,200 ORACs daily, the Tufts researchers recommend at least 3,500 ORACs daily and preferably between 5,000 and

---

Fresh Versus Frozen for Maximum Vitamin Content

Nothing against Mother Nature, but there are advantages to modern-day processing techniques when it comes to preserving the nutrients in produce, especially vegetables. Because the nutritional content of most vegetables begins to diminish the moment they're picked, and up to 2 weeks can pass by the time these foods make it to your local supermarket, they can have lost as much as 50 percent of their nutritional punch by the time they actually make it to your refrigerator. Frozen vegetables, by contrast, usually are processed relatively quickly after being picked and thus often will have a higher nutritional value by the time they make it to your plate. Because canned vegetables usually are partially cooked before being canned, however, and because large amounts of sodium (salt) are often added, these may not be a better choice than fresh. Remember, too, that most vegetables lose nutrients the longer they're cooked.

6,000 to play it extra safe.[18] If that sounds like a lot, it's not, as you'll see from the list. For example, a cup of blueberries with breakfast and an orange with lunch puts you at over 4,000 ORACs, and that's even before your spinach with dinner and fresh cantaloupe for dessert! See table 2. (*Note:* Fruits and vegetables are great sources of not only disease-fighting antioxidants but other important vitamins, minerals, and fiber as well.)

Table 2.   Antioxidant Potency of Fruits and Vegetables

Food	Antioxidant Potency (in ORACs)
Blueberries, 1/2 cup (fresh)	1,620
Blackberries, 1/2 cup (fresh)	1,466
Kale, 1/2 cup (cooked)	1,150
Strawberries, 1/2 cup (fresh)	1,144
Spinach, 1 cup (cooked)	1,089
Raisins, 1/4 cup	1,019
Orange, 1 medium	982
Cranberries, 1/2 cup (fresh)	831
Broccoli florets, 1/2 cup (cooked)	817
Raspberries, 1/2 cup (fresh)	755
Beets, 1/2 cup (cooked, sliced)	715
Cantaloupe, 1/2 melon	670
Beans, 1/2 cup (baked)	640
Plum, 1 medium	626
Grapefruit, pink, 1 medium	580
Pepper, red, 1 medium	540
Watermelon, 1 medium piece	501

Source: Adapted from G. Cao et al., "Increases in Human Plasma Antioxidant Capacity After Consumption of Controlled Diets in Fruits and Vegetables," *American Journal of Clinical Nutrition* 68, no. 5 (November 1998).

Other Good Sources

While the fruits and vegetables just listed are our best antioxidant sources, these other foods also should be included in your diet whenever possible: prunes, cherries, apples, grapes, peas, kidney beans, cauliflower, eggplant, potatoes, apricots, cabbage, brussels sprouts, kiwi-fruit, onions, garlic, carrots, yellow squash, zucchini, tomatoes, tofu, string beans, leaf lettuce, peaches, pears, bananas, and corn.

Consider Vitamin E

While not all experts agree on the amount of vitamin E needed to help protect against the development of Alzheimer's disease, few dispute its value. Most of the nutritionists we talked to who were familiar with the most current research on vitamin E and Alzheimer's recommended between 400 and 800 IUs daily—an amount well in excess of the 30 IUs that constitute the current Recommended Daily Value. However, Paul Raia, Ph.D., the director of patient care for the Alzheimer's Association in Cambridge, Massachusetts, advises daily doses higher than that—between 800 and 1,600 IUs—to help keep AD at bay. (All experts *do* agree, however, that it's important to get clearance from one's doctor before taking vitamin E supplements in any amount, as the vitamin may react adversely with some medications or cause bleeding or gastrointestinal problems in rare cases.)

The evidence for E? A study reported in the *New England Journal of Medicine* in 1997 found that people in moderate stages of Alzheimer's disease who were given large doses of vitamin E (2,000 IUs daily) experienced a significant slow-down in the development of certain symptoms, including loss of ability to do daily activities.[19] Scientists believe vitamin E works to help combat AD by functioning as an antioxidant, meaning it helps neutralize the harmful activity of molecules known as free radicals that damage cells—brain cells, especially—by disrupting their molecular structure.

Whether vitamin E can help prevent Alzheimer's disease from developing in the first place has yet to be determined, but many experts feel its benefits at this point far outweigh its risks. In the words of Mark Sager, M.D., for example, the director of the Wisconsin Alzheimer's Institute at the University of Wisconsin in Madison, "Because the pathological evidence of Alzheimer's disease may be present in the brain for many years prior to the development of symptoms, it is possible that vitamin E could delay the onset of, or even prevent the disease."[20]

> *Whether vitamin E can help prevent Alzheimer's disease from developing in the first place has yet to be determined, but many experts feel its benefits at this point far outweigh its risks.*

This point remains to be proven, Dr. Sager concedes, and currently it is the subject of a large national study—the Memory Impairment Study—being sponsored by the National Institute on Aging. Even before the results are in, however, Dr. Sager advocates that people who currently have AD should take between 1,000 and 2,000 IUs daily, encouraging persons who may be at increased risk for the disease (for example, family members) to take supplemental vitamin E as well. "Vitamin E is safe," Dr. Sager says, "and has multiple benefits, especially for the heart."[21]

Get Enough Folate

Another nutrient attracting attention for its ability to help prevent Alzheimer's disease in recent years has been folate, also called folic acid. Beginning in the late 1970s, researchers began noticing connections not only between low levels of folate and mothers giving birth to babies with brain defects but also between low folate levels and increased risks of brain atrophy (shrinkage) in the elderly. Most recently, this latter finding was replicated in the Nun Study by Dr. Snowdon, who found a definite link between low levels of folate in the blood and increased risks of brain atrophy typical of AD. "Since Alzheimer's can be viewed as a brain wasting disease," Dr. Snowdon says, "it is reasonable to think that folic acid deficiency could move the process of atrophy into high gear."[22]

Folate may exert its protective effects against AD by joining forces with vitamin B_{12} in breaking down a compound known as homocysteine, which scientists have found contributes to the buildup of plaque within the arteries—a process that could play role in the development of AD by compromising blood flow to the brain. Homocysteine also appears to be toxic to brain cells directly, however, "thus speeding the atrophy of the Alzheimer's brain," Dr. Snowdon says. In a recent study headed by British researcher Robert Clarke, Ph.D., for example, high levels of homocysteine in the blood were found to raise risks of Alzheimer's disease by a disturbing 450 percent,[23] results reinforced by a more recent 2002 study reported in the *New England Journal of Medicine*. (See sidebar, "Homocysteine.")

Dr. Snowdon found a definite link between low levels of folate in the blood and increased risks of brain atrophy typical of AD.

More definitive evidence of folate's protective effects against AD will be available in a few years with the completion of a large-scale study being sponsored by the National Institutes of Health, and Dr. Snowdon says he feels "particularly optimistic" about what this study will find. As for the amount of folate required to exert a protective effect against AD, most experts agree that the current Recommended Daily Value of 400 micrograms—the amount in most multiple-vitamin tablets— is sufficient to do the job.[24]

Stock an Anti-Alzheimer's Pantry

While research suggests we may be able to reduce our risks of Alzheimer's disease by keeping plenty of fruits and vegetables in our refrigerators, it appears we'd do well to keep some potent AD fighters stocked in our pantries, too.

Curry Powder

This common spice, due to the compound curcumin (also called cumin) prevalent in its principal ingredient, turmeric, may be able to perk up

Homocysteine

Homocysteine has been suspected of playing a role in the onset of Alzheimer's disease for some time, but perhaps never as convincingly as was demonstrated in a study reported in February of 2002 in the *New England Journal of Medicine*.[25] "Some of the most powerful evidence to date," is how the National Institutes of Health (NIH) chose to describe the investigation which tracked the health of 1,092 elderly people for a period of more than 20 years.[26] Those who were found to have high levels of homocysteine in their blood (defined as greater than 14 mmols/liter) proved to be twice as likely to have developed AD 20 years later as people whose levels had been normal. For each 5 mmols a person's homocysteine reading exceeded this level of 14, moreover, risks of developing AD increased by another 40 percent, suggesting a "more is worse" scenario.

brain activity as well as a good stew. Intrigued by studies showing that rates of Alzheimer's disease in India are the lowest in the world—1 percent of people 65 and older compared to 10 percent in the United States—Sally Frautschy, Ph.D., of the University of California at Los Angeles decided to see whether the potent antioxidant and anti-inflammatory curcumin might play a role. She fed a diet rich in curcumin to rats that had been genetically engineered to develop Alzheimer's disease. Sure enough, the animals experienced a reduction in inflammation of neurological tissue as well as a partial clearing of amyloid plaque from the synapses between nerve cells. The animals also were better able to negotiate a maze following their spicy diets, showing that the changes in their brains had been responsible for a significant improvement in their memories. Curcumin may not be the only brain-friendly spice in our racks, moreover, as Dr. Frautschy notes that rosemary and ginger contain compounds very similar to those in curcumin and hence should produce similar neurological effects.[27]

Some scientists have chosen to see a bright side to this discovery, however—Neil Buckholtz, Ph.D., of the National Institute on Aging, for example, says that "the good news is that we may have found a risk factor for AD that is modifiable."[28] Dr. Buckholtz is referring to research showing that vitamins B_6, B_{12}, and folate all have been shown to help keep homocysteine levels in check—so much so, in fact, that the National Institute on Aging recently embarked on a nationwide study to see if these nutrients might help arrest cases of Alzheimer's disease already in progress.

For those of us interested in AD prevention, moreover, it certainly can't hurt to be sure we're getting these nutrients in adequate amounts, most nutritionists agree. This can be done either through supplementation or a diet rich in green leafy vegetables, low-fat dairy products, citrus fruits and juices, whole wheat products, and dried beans, according to a recent NIH report.[29]

Tea

For a healthy dose of antioxidants with nary a calorie, tea is tops. According to an analysis of a wide variety of teas done by researchers at Tufts University, a 5-ounce cup of black or green tea serves up a whopping 1,246 ORAC units—which puts this courtly beverage right up there with such antioxidant powerhouses as strawberries and spinach. Black tea tends to be slightly higher in antioxidants than green, but only by about 20 percent, these researchers found. Most herbal teas were determined to contain relatively few antioxidants, while instant (powdered) and bottled teas also were found to have negligible amounts. Decaffeination? It reduces antioxidant levels by about 50 percent, according to the Tufts report.[30]

While green tea may lag slightly behind black tea in antioxidants overall, it contains four times as much of a particular type of antioxidant called *epigallocatechin gallate* (EGCG), which some researchers feel makes green tea the better choice for reducing AD risks. EGCG

Antioxidants: The Body's Heroes

If nutritional compounds could win Purple Hearts, antioxidants would have a chest full. These microscopic heroes sacrifice themselves thousands of times every second to protect us from not just Alzheimer's disease but also some 60 or more other health problems, ranging from heart disease to hemorrhoids.

To understand how antioxidants work, it helps to understand what they work against—molecules called free radicals that are created as natural by-products of many key metabolic processes within the body but that can be very harmful if not kept in check. A free radical is created when a normally stable molecule loses an electron, a fact of atomic life that causes the free radical to seek to replace this electron by stealing one from whatever other "healthy" molecule it may meet. This becomes a biochemical version of "robbing Peter to pay Paul," as the molecule being stolen from seeks to repeat the crime against some other molecule to compensate for its loss.

has been found to be especially effective at inhibiting angiogenesis, a process whereby new blood vessels form in areas of the brain damaged by AD's amyloid plaques. Until recently, this vascularization was thought to be beneficial for people with AD, but new studies being done by researchers at the Angiogenesis Foundation in Cambridge, Massachusetts, now suggest that the process may actually do more harm than good by contributing significantly to plaque buildup. Soy protein, these researchers say, is another potent source of angiogenesis-inhibiting compounds. (See chapter 8 for more on the angiogenesis process.)

Red Wine

While the Alzheimer's Association does not officially condone the consumption of alcoholic beverages to help prevent Alzheimer's dis-

But what's so important about a missing electron or two? Molecules lacking an electron function either poorly or not at all, thus damaging whatever tissue or organ this molecule may help comprise. In the case of heart disease, free radicals are suspected of damaging cells that make up blood vessel walls, thus contributing to the buildup of artery-clogging plaque. Free radical damage to the cartilage within joints is thought to be a key factor in the development of arthritis. With respect to Alzheimer's disease, free radicals are believed to lead to the death of brain cells and the subsequent formation of AD's amyloid plaques.

Antioxidants to the rescue. Antioxidants have the unique ability to offer up electrons to appease these free radicals, but without in turn becoming part of the destructive free radical chain. The body is capable of producing some antioxidant compounds of its own, but it relies mostly on antioxidants in the foods we eat. Fruits and vegetables generally offer the most antioxidants, but many other foods, beverages, and supplements also can be great sources.

ease, it does acknowledge "a possible relationship between moderate consumption of wine and a reduced risk."[31] This concession comes based on substantial research, including one study done in 1997 of more than 3,600 people over the age of 65 living in Bordeaux, France, where 97 percent of the alcohol consumed is in the form of wine, most of it red. The study was reported at a meeting of the American Academy of Neurology in 1997, and its results undeniably were worth toasting. Moderate drinkers—defined by the French researchers as those averaging three to four glasses of wine daily—were found to be only 25 percent as likely to develop Alzheimer's disease as people who didn't drink at all. This protective effect was lost, however, in people whose consumption was more excessive, suggesting there's a point of diminishing returns regarding the healthful effects of alcohol that we all would do well to heed.

Why might red wine be protective against AD? It's a great source of antioxidants, which are thought to come from the skins of the grapes from which it's made. Then, too, moderate drinking of any type of alcoholic beverage appears to help protect against strokes, which are a known AD risk. Remember, however, that moderation is key. Research shows that heavy drinking can harm virtually every organ of the body—the brain included.

> *As mentioned earlier, the Nun Study has found that the antioxidant lycopene seems to be uniquely protective against mental impairment as we age.*

Tomato Products

As mentioned earlier, the Nun Study has found that the antioxidant lycopene seems to be uniquely protective against mental impairment as we age. In eight women between the ages of 77 and 98, Dr. Snowdon found that those with the highest levels of lycopene in their blood were four times less likely to need assistance with such activities as walking, dressing, bathing, and feeding themselves as women whose lycopene levels were the lowest.[32] In *Your Miracle Brain*, Jean Carper reports an Italian study in which people who ate 16.5 milligrams of lycopene daily in the form of tomato paste for just 3 weeks were able to boost the antioxidant levels in their blood enough to reduce the damaging activity of free radicals by a remarkable 33 percent.[33]

Contrary to the notion that "fresh is best," researchers have found that products made from cooked rather than fresh tomatoes seem to be our best lycopene sources, which certainly puts a new spin on the likes of spaghetti sauce and ketchup. The best sources of this potent antioxidant are listed in table 3.

Dried Fruits, Jellies, and Jams

Dried fruits may be a more concentrated source of calories than fresh, but they also are a more concentrated source of brain-friendly antioxidants. Just a quarter cup of raisins, for example, has over 1,000 ORACs of antioxidant firepower (almost a third of what nutritionists

Table 3.   Sources of Lycopene

Food	Lycopene per Ounce (in milligrams)
Tomato paste	16
Tomato ketchup	5
Spaghetti sauce	5
Tomato sauce	5
Tomato soup	3
Tomato juice	3
Vegetable juice	3
Tomatoes, canned	3
Tomatoes, fresh	1
Grapefruit, pink	1
Watermelon	1

Source: Adapted from Jean Carper, *Your Miracle Brain* (New York: HarperCollins, 2000).

now recommend), and just three prunes provide a hefty 1,386 ORACs. Other dried fruits such as apricots, apples, bananas, and pears are not as bountiful with antioxidants as prunes and raisins, but they still are worthwhile sources. Jellies and jams? If they're made from real fruit instead of mostly corn syrup or sugar, these can be great antioxidant sources, too.

Treat Your Brain to the Most Brain-Friendly Fats

What role might dietary fat play in the onset of Alzheimer's disease? Research is preliminary but very intriguing. Some scientists believe the type of dietary fat we eat can affect our brains profoundly, influencing not just our risks of developing Alzheimer's disease but even our ability to function day to day. In *Your Miracle Brain*, Carper summarizes this

AD and the Environment: Meddling Metals?

Should we be concerned about toxins in the environment as Alzheimer's risks? "There are several theories about environmental triggers for AD, but no one trigger has been clearly identified," reports the education director at the Mather Institute on Aging and author of *Alzheimer's Early Stages,* Daniel Kuhn, M.S.W.[34]

Fears that aluminum might cause AD surfaced back in 1965 when injections of aluminum salts into the brains of rabbits were found to produce brain damage that resembled Alzheimer's disease in humans, but subsequent research showed that the damage was not the same after all. Aluminum was further exonerated in the 1980s when studies refuted earlier evidence that Alzheimer's disease might be caused by high levels of aluminum in drinking water. This is not to deny that aluminum has neurotoxic properties that can be harmful for patients who must receive huge amounts of the metal when undergoing dialysis for kidney failure, but these amounts exceed normal levels of exposure by fifty-fold, notes University of Kentucky professor of neurology and director of the Nun Study, David Snowdon, Ph.D. "To date, most Alzheimer's researchers, myself in-

research by calling the type of fat we eat "one of the most critical decisions" regarding the health of our brains that we can make.[35]

The most healthful fats, Carper reports, are monounsaturated fats (prevalent in olive oil and nuts), which have antioxidant properties similar to those of fruits and vegetables. Also brain-friendly is a type of polyunsaturated fat, omega-3, found most commonly in cold-water fish such as mackerel and salmon. This type of fat has been shown to help neutralize free radical activity, fight inflammation, aid the action of neurotransmitters, and even help brain cells maintain their basic structure.

The fats to be avoided are the saturated kind found predominantly in animal foods such as meat, whole milk, butter, and cheese, cluded, have been unconvinced by the evidence against aluminum," he says.[36]

Also unconvincing in recent years has been evidence that the mercury from silver amalgam fillings once used in dentistry might increase AD risks. This scare was ignited by the influential TV show *60 Minutes* in 1990, but Dr. Snowdon reports that studies since then, including his own Nun Study, have determined that mercury from dental fillings does not pose an AD threat. Also absolved in recent years have been iron and zinc, although, as Kuhn notes, "There still may be unidentified chemicals or other toxic substances in the environment that play a role in AD's development."[37]

Such substances that have been identified, Kuhn says, are organic solvents such as benzene and toluene. A study in Canada has found that people whose jobs expose them to high levels of certain pesticides, fertilizers, and glue also may be at increased risk.[38] There also is evidence from one small study that exposures to electromagnetic fields (e.g., those produced by high-tension electrical wires) may elevate risks of AD,[39] but Kuhn says these results should in no way be considered conclusive until more research is done.

researchers say. In addition to increasing risks for heart disease, these fats have been shown in studies by Carol E. Greenwood, Ph.D., of the University of Toronto, to impair the learning ability of laboratory animals.[40] Also to be limited is the omega-6 type of polyunsaturated fat prevalent in certain vegetable oils (discussed later) that some research suggests may be unhealthy for brain cells by causing inflammation as well by creating free radicals when metabolized. Hydrogenated fats, made by adding hydrogen to saturated fat, and prevalent in many baked goods and snack foods, also may trigger cell malformation that's bad for the brain, Carper reports.[41]

When it comes time to make a salad or fry some fish, Carper offers these tips:

- Avoid oils highest in omega-6 fatty acids, such as safflower, sunflower, and corn, and avoid using margarines, mayonnaise, and salad dressings made predominantly from these oils as well. Also limit your intake of snack foods that contain hydrogenated fats such as chips, crackers, and popcorn, and avoid margarines, mayonnaise, and salad dressings that contain hydrogenated fats, too.

- Try to use oils rich in omega-3 fatty acids whenever possible; these include flaxseed oil (the richest of all in omega-3s), canola, and peanut. Olive oil also is a healthful choice for being

---

Brain Abuse

In *Your Miracle Brain,* esteemed health journalist Jean Carper, who also wrote the *New York Times* bestseller *Miracle Cures,* contends that as a nation, we're treating our brains as if they were our arch enemies rather than critical allies. The crimes we commit routinely in the course of our daily lives, she says, include the following:

- We eat the wrong types of fats "guaranteed to cause disruption in the functioning of our brains, perhaps ending in neuronal death."

- We eat too much sugar, "dumping excessive glucose into the brain where it reacts with free radicals to literally burn brain cells to death."

- We overeat, creating a calorie overload that produces even more free radicals destined to "condemn brain cells to dysfunction and death."

- We skimp on eating fresh fruits and vegetables, our best sources of antioxidants capable of defending against such carnage by putting free radicals under arrest.

a great source of monounsaturated fat, which researchers are finding to be beneficial for the heart.

- Try to eat fish high in omega-3s, such as salmon, mackerel, herring, sardines, anchovies, bluefin tuna, whitefish, and trout.

Protect Your Brain from High Blood Pressure and Cholesterol

Doctors have suspected for some time that high blood pressure and high cholesterol levels might increase risks of Alzheimer's disease, and

- We "cheat ourselves of precious nutrients such as B vitamins and vitamin E, essential for good mental function."
- We do "subtle but serious damage" to our brains by enduring high blood pressure, high cholesterol levels, and insulin resistance characteristic of diabetes.
- We shun exercise, which is a proven energizer of brain activity and a staunch defender against depression.
- We cheat our brains of the mental activity needed to keep them healthy by spending hours a day in front of the television and allowing our children to do the same.[42]

It's a wonder we can spell our names given the picture Carper paints, but we shouldn't allow her powerful words to obscure the basic truth in what she says. Many of us do treat our brains poorly and may be increasing our risks for Alzheimer's and other dementias in the process.

recently they got some eye-opening proof. A study of over 1,400 people, completed in June 2001 and reported in the *British Medical Journal*, found that people who had either high blood pressure or high cholesterol in their 40s and 50s—and failed to do anything about it over the next 21 years—had increased their risks of developing AD by over 200 percent. While people with high blood pressure (defined as systolic readings of 160 or greater) were 2.3 times more likely to develop AD, those with high cholesterol levels (250 milligrams/deciliter or higher) were 2.1 times more prone. Having both conditions, not surprisingly, increased risks even more—to 3.5 times above normal.[43]

> *Doctors have suspected for some time that high blood pressure and high cholesterol levels might increase risks of Alzheimer's disease.*

These elevated risks held up, moreover, even after other potentially confounding lifestyle factors such as smoking, obesity, and alcohol consumption were taken into consideration. Commenting on the study, Steve Seiner, M.D., an instructor of psychiatry at Harvard Medical School, said the results should send out an important message to all of us that seeds of Alzheimer's disease may get sown long before the illness finally appears. "We need to take care of our bodies and our basic health when we're younger in order to help lower our risk for Alzheimer's disease later in life," he said.[44]

Regarding the role cholesterol may play in the development of AD, some studies suggest that high levels may work in the brain directly to add to the buildup of amyloid plaque. Studies with rodents, for example, have shown that diets high in cholesterol lead to greater plaque accumulation, which drugs that lower cholesterol then help reduce. The suspicion is that high cholesterol levels may contribute to the formation of a protein thought to play a key role in plaque formation, says Rudolph Tanzi, Ph.D., professor of neurology at Harvard Medical School and the author of *Decoding Darkness: The Search for Genetic Causes of Alzheimer's Disease*. Dr. Tanzi has issued warnings that are even more specific. "We're seeing more and more that what's bad for the heart is bad for the brain," he says. "With any risk factor linked to heart disease, you need to pay attention to it for Alzheimer's as well."[45]

As we'll be seeing in chapter 8, further support that AD might have a cholesterol connection comes from research showing that people who take drugs called *statins* to lower high cholesterol levels seem to gain significant protection from the disease. In one such study of over 60,000 people reported in the *Archives of Neurology*, researchers from the Loyola University Medical Center outside Chicago found that people who had been taking either of two statins for lowering cholesterol (lovastatin or pravastatin) had reduced their risks of developing Alzheimer's disease by 60 to 70 percent.[46]

> *We're seeing more and more that what's bad for the heart is bad for the brain.*
>
> —RUDOLPH TANZI, PH.D.

Further evidence of a cholesterol-Alzheimer's link has been suggested by a study in which mice genetically engineered to have Alzheimer's disease experienced an increase in both the size and number of their beta-amyloid plaques when fed a high-cholesterol diet.[47] Much more research needs to be done to determine the precise nature of the cholesterol-Alzheimer's connection, but it's an area of great interest that many researchers agree could produce an important breakthrough.

CHAPTER 8

Racing for a Cure

✍

T HE RACE FOR a cure to Alzheimer's disease is on, with many entrepreneurial feet running flat out and government funds providing a boost. But AD's clock ticks toward trying times: As mentioned previously, scientists estimate 4 million Americans already suffer from the disease, with 360,000 new victims adding to the carnage each year. Ominously, the incidence of Alzheimer's doubles every 5 years among people over 65. Today, an estimated 35 million Americans are 65 or older; according to the U.S. Bureau of the Census, that number will have doubled to 70 million by 2050. A shifting balance between working and retired Americans compounds the problem. As the baby-boomer bulge in our population begins to reach 65 in fewer than 10 years, the number of workers relative to retirees will start to decline, reducing per capita resources for the aged.

These numbers are mind numbing, even for today's most alert brains. Current medical costs for managing AD range up to $100 billion annually in the United States. As a result of our aging population, the number of victims could rise to 14 million in the United States alone by the middle of this century. When we factor in an average life expectancy of 8 years subsequent to diagnosis and multiply some portion of that time by the Alzheimer's Association's estimate of $42,000 annually for nursing home care of one victim with severe cognitive impairment, the projected cost is staggering. It's safe to say AD will put a devastating financial dent in the economies of developed countries until a cure is found.

SAME TARGET, SEPARATE GOALS

The federal government, charitable organizations, the medical and scientific communities, as well as private firms have all joined the war in an effort to defeat Alzheimer's. A cure can both save and make big dollars. Unlike rare diseases, normally ignored by pharmaceutical companies due to a low return on investment, AD offers a potential financial bonanza. "My CEO said it's costing us $150,000 a day not to have an Alzheimer's drug on the market," revealed a researcher for one company.[1]

For current and prospective victims of the disease, the far-ranging research is encouraging news. The affliction is widespread and growing, and it offers enormous profit potential in cultures most capable of paying the doctor's bill. Be assured, the giving and the greedy are both hard at work, though not always in concert.

COMPETITION: IS IT HELPFUL?

The profit potential and resultant secrecy clouding private AD research became evident at a major scientific conference in the early 1990s. During the gathering, Elan's head of research and development, Ivan Lieberburg, made the following celebratory announcement regarding his company's progress on Alzheimer's: "We're really on the threshold of a new age. I think we're coming very close to the goal line now."[2]

Following the conference, Lieberburg turned to David Shenk, author of *The Forgetting*, and confessed, "This was one of the most frustrating experiences I've ever had in my life, to speak to a group like this and not tell them what I know."[3]

While Allen Roses, a researcher for pharmaceutical giant Glaxo Wellcome, expresses similar concerns about secrecy, as well the possibility of intercompany espionage, he still feels that free enterprise fuels the fastest cures, citing diabetes as an example.[4]

Dr. William W. Li, M.D., a clinical instructor in medicine at Harvard Medical School and president and medical director of the Angiogenesis Foundation in Cambridge, Massachusetts, takes a broader perspective. He thinks that secrecy between companies chasing the same medical markets constitutes only part of the problem. Another major hindrance to progress, he says, is the lack of communication between scientific and medical specialists in various fields. "Today, we work in vertical silos," he explains. "Experts in oncology, neurology, endocrinology—you name it—constantly uncover new material that could be invaluable to a peer in another department just down the hall. But because so much work is done in isolation, critical discoveries often move slowly between specialties. To conquer Alzheimer's and other complex human afflictions, we have to speed up the cross-pollination of information between disciplines."

To draw an analogy, imagine the world's most brilliant human being, left alone on this planet, trying to build a modern bicycle. Just to locate iron and rubber, our genius would need geological and horticultural knowledge. Next would come mining, smelting, vulcanizing, casting, forging, machining, and so forth. Even if our mastermind were to get this far, an air pump for the tires would be a nice addition to make the bike functional. As the astronomer needs a lens maker, so must the surgeon have a scalpel. Suffice it to say that human progress is based on community effort.

> The World Wide Web will be a key catalyst in tackling Alzheimer's because it pulls patients, caregivers, physicians, researchers, governments, and private enterprises onto a smaller playing field where information can be shared more fruitfully and expeditiously.

As the complexity of human undertakings increases, so must the size of the information and technology bases on which these efforts depend for success. From Dr. Li's perspective, the World Wide Web will be a key catalyst in tackling Alzheimer's because it pulls patients, caregivers, physicians, researchers, governments, and private enterprises onto a smaller playing field where information can be shared more fruitfully and expeditiously.

FUNDING

Formed in 1974, the National Institute on Aging (NIA) soon targeted AD as a top priority, with research funding climbing from $13 million to over $75 million between 1980 and 1987. Then, following identification of a gene related to early-onset Alzheimer's, NIH's contribution grew even faster, to over $275 million by 1992. As of 2000, federal funding for AD research hovered in the $400 million range.

These numbers may represent only the tip of the iceberg for funding Alzheimer's research when we consider the investments being made by major pharmaceutical companies around the world whose goal is to tap an already-enormous and continually expanding market for treatments and cures. "By the year 2005 or 2010 the market could approach $8 billion," according to Kevin Felsenstein, a representative of Bristol-Myers Squibb. "If anything is going to define what a megablockbuster is, I think this would."[5]

FINDING THE TARGET

Within the research community, the cause of Alzheimer's engenders roiling debate. For example, early onset of the disease is relatively rare, affecting only 5 to 10 percent of people with AD and traceable to inherited defects on a small number of genes.[6] Later-onset AD presents a more complex problem, quite possibly linked not only to a broad spectrum of genetic factors but to environmental influences as well. Researchers continue to dispute whether the early and late manifestations are related. Some say they are two distinct diseases.

At the same time, camps have formed for and against the "beta-amyloid hypothesis"—most for, many fewer against. The theory proposes that tiny fragments snipped from amyloid precursor protein either directly damage brain cells or trigger a cascade of harmful events through which these fragments combine with remnants of nerve and supporting cells to create amyloid plaque.

Poor protein barbering appears to initiate the destructive process. When a beta-secretase enzyme rather than an alpha-secretase enzyme makes the first cut on the amyloid-precursor protein (which normally grows like a piece of hair from the membrane covering each brain cell), a second "enzyme barber," known as gamma secretase, makes its cut in the wrong place, leaving behind beta-amyloid peptides, the dangerous fragments.[7]

> *Within the research community, the cause of Alzheimer's engenders roiling debate.*

According to Steve Estus of the University of Kentucky in Lexington, a proponent of the theory, "The amyloid hypothesis is the simplest explanation possible." He goes on to suggest opponents of the idea do not see the whole picture provided by current evidence.[8] Indeed, beta amyloid can be toxic all by itself, as demonstrated in test-lab cultures where some forms produce free radicals that damage nerve cells. Likewise, plaques resulting from beta-amyloid have been tied to swelling and inflammation, possible harbingers of nerve cell death.[9]

While accepting the amyloid hypothesis as by far the most popular, John Blass, M.D., Ph.D., of Cornell University–Weill Medical College in New York says, "Looking at the same data, either you can see the doughnut, or you can see what to some of us looks like a very big hole."[10]

Some of the objections Dr. Blass and his supporters raise include the so-called 20/50 dilemma: At autopsy, 20 percent of people diagnosed with Alzheimer's have no beta-amyloid plaques in their brains. Conversely, 50 percent of autopsies performed on humans with no signs of cognitive impairment prior to death show relatively high amounts of beta-amyloid plaques in their brains. Stephen R. Robinson of Monash University in Clatyon, Australia, sums up the conundrum: "If one has a loose-fitting shoe, one will often see a blister. This doesn't mean the blister caused the loose-fitting shoe."[11]

Supporters of the beta-amyloid hypothesis explain these discrepancies by proposing that people with dementia but no plaques probably suffer from a type of mental decline other than Alzheimer's. Concerning people who were alert prior to death but showed plaques at autopsy, the counterargument contends that extra innate mental capacity in the form of larger brains or additional neural connections holds the disease at bay.[12]

Putting academic squabbles aside, the majority of researchers from both camps are excited by what they consider the true test of

BAPtists, Tauists, and Others

Brain tissues from Alzheimer's victims typically share two common features: beta-amyloid protein (BAP) and tau tangles. Which abnormality—if either—causes the disease fosters heated debate among researchers, who fall into three loosely defined camps: the BAPtists (supporters of the beta-amyloid hypothesis), Tauists (believers in tau tangles as the key culprit), and the others, whose speculations vary widely.

The BAPtists are already experimenting with approaches to inhibiting the formation of beta-amyloid and preventing, slowing, stopping, or reversing plaque buildup.

Tauists have succeeded in tracing abnormalities in tau proteins to some forms of dementia, but not yet to Alzheimer's. Nevertheless, investigations proceed to determine whether phosphorylated tau proteins, instead of tangles, might contribute to the disease.

whether beta-amyloid deposits cause Alzheimer's disease. Can inhibiting its formation and preventing the buildup of plaques stop the progression of the disease?

BEATING BETA-AMYLOID

Many major players in the pharmaceutical community—including Dupont, Merck, Elan, and Eli Lilly—have placed their bets on beta-amyloid as the most likely cause of Alzheimer's disease. At the same time (and this should come as good news), these companies are tackling the culprit from more than one side.

Alpha, *beta*, and *gamma* are "Greek" to most of us, but these descriptive tags are now used by researchers to describe three "brain

Michael Hutton at the Mayo Clinic in Jacksonville, Florida, takes an ecumenical approach. By inbreeding mice with mutated human genes for both the plaque and the tau, he has created progeny with more plaque and tau tangles than their ancestors, particularly in a region of the brain closely associated with memory.[13] These "doubly dumb" mice could play an important role in future experiments.

Another researcher straddling the fence, Peter Davies of the Albert Einstein College of Medicine in New York, showed that a Pin-1 protein not only binds to both the tau and amyloid precursor proteins but also returns phosphorylated tau proteins (bad guys) to a healthy state in the test tube. That's good news for human brains. On the negative side, Pin-1 may accelerate the formation of amyloid precursor protein because it contributes to cell division. Back to the positive perspective, Pin-1 could provide an epiphany, a revelation shared gladly in both the BAPtist and Tauist camps, by establishing a fundamental connection between plaque and tau tangles.[14]

barbers" (the enzymes alpha-secretase, beta-secretase, and gamma-secretase) that, according to one theory, produce neuron-destroying fibrils and plaques when they get their styling orders wrong (see figure 8.1).

Finding these "barbers" wasn't easy. But they have now been tracked down by biologists such as Bob Vassar, whose mother died at the age of 78 after living with Alzheimer's for 17 years. Working with Amgen, a major company in the field of biotechnology, Vassar designed a program through which 860,000 gene copies were tested to isolate beta-secretase, a "bad barber" enzyme. This discovery, also made at about the same time in 1999 by three other drug companies, presented exciting possibilities. As Lennart Mucke, director of the Gladstone Institute of Neurological Disease at the University of California, San Francisco, said, "It's a huge leap forward."[15] Indeed, it might be!

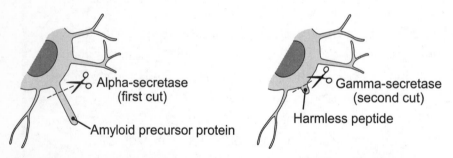

In normal cellular metabolism within the brain, amyloid precursor proteins are "clipped" by enzymes in a way that allows the clippings to harmlessly dissolve.

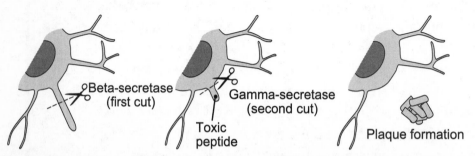

In the Alzheimer's brain, this process goes awry when the first cut is made by beta-secretase enzymes (instead of alpha-secretase) allowing the clippings to develop into harmful deposits known as amyloid plaques.

Figure 8.1—*Plaque Formation*

Stepping back for a moment, let's remember that drugs normally work like pieces in a three-dimensional jigsaw puzzle. They can be designed to encourage or discourage molecular fits. By slipping precisely into the grooves of a "bad barber" such as beta-secretase, a drug can neutralize its effects. In essence, the puzzle won't come together—or mutate—in the way the bad barber had planned. The threatening molecules are smoothed into the equivalent of spheres, obvious misfits, that our bodies flush away in the normal course of housecleaning.

> *By slipping precisely into the grooves of a "bad barber" such as beta-secretase, a drug can neutralize its effects.*

Along these lines, Amgen has mapped the three-dimensional structure of beta-secretase and plans to develop molecules capable of negating beta's plaque-building propensities. Other companies are charging down the same track. Elan Corporation, along with its partner, Pharmacia, is optimistic. "Both of us view beta-secretase as a terrific target," reports Dale Schenk, vice president of discovery research for Elan. "I don't think it's going to be terribly long before the field has clinical candidates."[16]

The history of AIDS research supports Schenk's positive outlook. The HIV protease, also an enzyme that cuts proteins and is presumed to be the cause of AIDS, was uncovered in 1989. After determining its structure, drug companies required fewer than 3 years to develop countermeasures for clinical trial. Today, the resulting drugs make a major contribution to the longevity and well-being of people with AIDS. The disease, in most cases, can now be controlled. It's no longer an automatic marching order to the gallows.[17]

When Bristol-Myers Squibb began the first known human trials on a secretase inhibitor designed to combat beta-amyloid, the protein fragment associated with Alzheimer's, Kevin Felsenstein, who heads the company's research program, announced, "We're on the verge now of either preventing amyloid deposits from building up, inhibiting the production of amyloid, or actually being able to reverse plaque deposition."[18] If beta-amyloid is the problem, that's great news.

A VACCINATION FOR ALZHEIMER'S?

Possibly more encouraging is a novel approach conceived by Elan's Dale Schenk. The idea is so simple that it seemed silly at the time. Why not just inject beta-amyloid peptide, the assumed cause of brain plaque, into transgenic mice (the creatures genetically engineered to accrue plaque) as a vaccination against plaque formation? That way the mice's own immune systems would be stimulated to perform a potentially therapeutic brain cleanup. Alzheimer's researcher Huntington Potter admits, "It's almost an obvious experiment, but we all assumed it would be a bad thing to do."[19]

Within his own company, Schenk faced stalwart skepticism. Nevertheless, his persistence paid off with amazing results reported throughout the media in 1999. Vaccinating the mice with beta-amyloid peptide prevented the formation of amyloid plaques. In one group of mice immunized at 6 weeks (an age well before plaque normally appears), the brains remained clean when inspected at 13 months, whereas nonimmunized mice with the same genetic makeup showed no reduction in plaque formation. Possibly more exciting were the results on mice who had been immunized at 11 months after plaque had already formed. Seven months later, these immunized 18-month-olds demonstrated significantly less plaque than their untreated peers of the same age but also less than untreated mice 6 months younger. The data suggested plaque formation could not only be prevented but reversed as well. Commenting on a second study in which mice were vaccinated, Schenk reported, "The absence of subsequent neuronal degenerative and related inflammatory changes that usually occur around amyloid plaque suggests that treated mice never developed the degenerative lesions associated with Alzheimer's disease."[20]

Independent results published by researchers in December 2000 held out additional promise, if not for a cure, then at least for a treatment. Again, mice genetically altered to form plaque were vaccinated, but in this case, a new dimension was added—measurements of memory. Although the overall performance of the vaccinated mice in water maze tests was not up to that of "normal" mice in the study, it was significantly better than that of transgenic mice who had not received the vaccine.[21]

As a next step in bringing a vaccine to market, Elan and Wyeth-Ayerst Laboratories, the pharmaceutical division of American Home Products, commenced clinical trials on humans in January 2000. In July 2001, Elan reported that in phase 1 human safety studies, its experimental treatment known as AN-1792 had been administered in a variety of dosage regimens to more than 100 people with mild to moderate Alzheimer's and that the treatment was well tolerated, meaning it caused no serious side effects.[22] "More importantly," explained Ivan Lieberburg, executive vice president and chief science and medical officer of Elan, "we saw that in a significant proportion of the patients, they were able to demonstrate an immune response. Their antibody levels went up and that indicates that this was having an effect in these patients."[23]

> *Vaccinating the mice with beta-amyloid peptide prevented the formation of amyloid plaques. . . . The data suggested plaque formation could not only be prevented but reversed as well.*

A Setback

For reasons not yet fully understood, Elan's vaccine suffered a serious setback when some of its recipients began developing brain inflammation during phase 2 of its clinical trial, causing the study to be discontinued, but experts stress that the basic concept behind the vaccine remains sound and will continue to be explored. "The failure of the vaccine in no way dampens enthusiasm for the amyloid hypothesis," notes Rudolph Tanzi, Ph.D., the author of *Decoding Darkness* and professor of neurology at Harvard Medical School and the director of the Massachusetts General Hospital's Genetics and Aging Unit. "The future of the vaccine may now have to be one of passive immunization, whereby antibodies will need to be raised in the lab and then injected as opposed to allowing the body itself to be the antibody producer," Dr. Tanzi says. (For updates on Elan's progress, visit its Web site at www.elan.com.)

Phases 1, 2, and 3 in Testing Drugs: What Do They Mean?

All three of these phases in testing drugs are conducted using human subjects. Phase 1 determines whether a drug is safe and in what dosages. Phase 2 tries to determine *efficacy*—that is, whether the drug performs its intended function. Phase 3 normally includes a larger number of subjects to further test safety and efficacy, as well as produce data for evaluation by the Food and Drug Administration (FDA). Normally, drugs are not tested on humans before being evaluated in animal tests.

RESURRECTING THE BRAIN

Once we've lost some brain power, can it come back? Many researches say yes.

Consider a drug in phase 3 clinical trials as of December 2001, developed by NeoTherapeutics, a company based in Irvine, California. Called Neotrofin, the drug presents possibilities for regrowing neurons, the cells enabling us to think. As detailed by Eve Taylor, Ph.D., director of biomolecular pharmacology at NeoTherapeutics, "A single dose of Neotrofin reproducibly results in a statistically significant increase in the number of stem cells in the brains of adult mice." She added, "We have now completed the analysis of two studies on differentiation of these neural stem cells. . . . We observed statistically significant increases in the number of new neurons 6 weeks after a single treatment with Neotrofin."[24]

Neotrofin is presumed to work in a double-faceted fashion through which communication between neurons is improved and stem cells, capable of producing new neurons, proliferate. In December 2001, a spokesperson for the company said:

We are now in phase 3 trials. During phase 2 trials, we saw compelling case-history indications that the drug may not only stop, but also reverse the effects of Alzheimer's disease. A dear older woman, previously a bookkeeper who motored around quite nicely before being afflicted with Alzheimer's, was one of the subjects. She could no longer drive or get her numbers right when she came into the phase 2 trial. During the course of the trial, she regained her ability to drive and keep the ledgers straight. Sadly, she declined after the trial when the experimental treatment with Neotrofin stopped. She's not alone.

NeoTherapeutics anticipates filing for FDA approval of Neotrofin for "symptomatic" relief of Alzheimer's by the end of 2002 or early 2003. Concurrently, the company will press forward with phase 3 studies to gain FDA acceptance of Neotrofin as a "disease-modifying" drug—that is, one that treats the disease, not just the symptoms. Updates about Neotrofin should be available at www.neot.com.

Another approach to rebuilding brains ravaged by Alzheimer's is the direct introduction of stem cells from which fresh neurons can grow. Putting political controversy over stem cell research aside for a moment, many scientists argue that any cells bred from a gene stock other than that of the recipient won't blend into the body smoothly; instead, they will be rejected as "aliens." Robert Lanza—nurtured by really big-leaguers such as psychologist B. F. Skinner, polio stopper Jonas Salk, and heart transplant vanguard Christian Barnard—worked for two decades on curing people with diabetes and leukemia by introducing replacement organs and cells from donors. "For twenty years, I hit my head against the same thing over and over again—rejection, rejection, rejection," said Lanza.[25] Using drugs to prevent rejection often backfired.

The seemingly simple, but in actuality not so simple, answer comes down to human cloning—making a duplicate of one's self so replacement

> *Another approach to rebuilding brains ravaged by Alzheimer's is the direct introduction of stem cells from which fresh neurons can grow.*

A Mental Tune-Up?

We all run out of gas on occasion and, as a result, typically slow down until making a pit stop for fuel (food containing glucose). However, when fatigue is chronic, as in the case of people with diabetes, the problem is usually a misfiring engine, not just a low gas tank. Diabetics have difficulty converting glucose into energy.

So, too, may people with Alzheimer's, postulates John Blass, M.D., Ph.D., of Cornell University–Weill Medical College. Measurements on both humans and animals show that a drop in brain metabolism usually leads to a decline in cognitive function. While suggesting that the plaques and tangles seen in Alzheimer's could

parts fit perfectly. While this idea is almost universally objectionable from a macroscopic perspective ("Breed another me so I can harvest replacement parts"), it seems much more palatable on a cellular scale ("Get another me started in a petri dish so I can be infused with my fresh cells"). As most experts point out, the new cells might give us some breathing space, but if not corrected at the genetic level, they will eventually produce the same problems with which we started. Nevertheless, human cloning could offer a reprieve for victims of Alzheimer's, and, when combined with genetic manipulations, the fix might stick. "In the meantime," reports *Scientific American*, "a lot of sick people who have read the headlines [about stem cell research] are pinning their hopes on this potentially revolutionary course of treatment. Without cloning, [these methods] aren't likely to work."[26]

ANTI-ANGIOGENESIS: FIXING RESCUE EFFORTS GONE WRONG

"Discovery consists of seeing what everybody else has been seeing but thinking what nobody else has thought."

either be caused by or result from poor brain metabolism, Dr. Blass proposed boosting mental energy as a method of treatment.

To test this idea, a drink containing sugar and malate, a compound that tunes up cellular engines (mitochondria), was given daily to seven people with Alzheimer's. Over 3 months, all seven showed improvement on standard mental tests, according to Dr. Blass. As a consequence of these positive results, Dr. Blass and his colleagues planned a larger study in which some subjects will receive a placebo and others the brain-boosting cocktail. To minimize the possibility of wishful thinking clouding results, neither the human subjects nor the physicians evaluating them will know who received the real cocktail and who didn't.[27]

That remark by Nobel Prize–winner Albert Szent-Gyorgi characterizes the thinking behind what could be "a major breakthrough in our understanding and treatment, not just of Alzheimer's, but possibly some other major illnesses as well," says Dr. Li. Working with Anthony H. Vagnucci, Jr., M.D., of Cambridge (Massachusetts) Hospital, Dr. Li has come up with a new way of looking at a basic physiological process that scientists have known about for years but that has not been considered as contributing to Alzheimer's disease. Called *angiogenesis*, the process is important in the body, but Drs. Li and Vagnucci have reason to believe that in Alzheimer's disease, this "friend" may instead be a serious "foe."

"Angiogenesis is the body's way of trying to rescue injured tissue, which it does by promoting the growth of new blood vessels for the purpose of bringing oxygen and nutrients to the area of injury to initiate repair," Dr. Li explains. "It occurs anywhere blood flow needs improvement, not only in the elderly brain but also in conditions such as heart attacks and strokes where circulation is seriously compromised, and angiogenesis can be a veritable lifesaver by restoring lost blood flow. It's well known that Alzheimer's brains could use more circulation."

Our Genes: A Stacked Deck

Many of the noninfectious diseases we encounter in our lives are, to a large degree, determined by our genetic makeup. For example, early-onset AD, affecting people in the age range of 30 to 60 years, is relatively rare, runs in families, and is traceable to a small number of genes. Later-onset AD, in contrast, presents a much murkier picture. Although evidence from genetic and epidemiological studies suggest an inherited proclivity for late-onset Alzheimer's, the disease's mechanism is complex and unpredictable. Even in identical twins, AD can emerge in one twin a decade or more before or after being observed in the other twin, or not at all.

Likewise, late onset may be triggered by a combination of minor genetic flaws that only begin to manifest themselves with age.[28] The APOE gene, when inherited in a form known as ApoE4, for instance, can move up the onset of Alzheimer's by as much as 17 years.[29] In fact, a commercial test for the presence of ApoE4 is now available but normally recommended only as an aid in differentiating Alz-

As well intended as angiogenesis is, however, in the brains of people with Alzheimer's disease, the process goes dangerously wrong. Cells that make up the newly formed blood vessels in people with AD react to free radicals given off by AD's amyloid plaques in a way that makes them contribute to the very problem the blood vessels had been formed to correct.

"The situation becomes a kind of molecular catch-22," Dr. Li says. "Free radicals emitted by the amyloid plaque cause the blood vessels to become sticky and attract a substance called *thrombin*, which in turn causes the blood vessels to release molecules that turn into more amyloid plaque. This plaque in turn produces more free radicals, which cause the production of more thrombin, which leads to more plaque."

heimer's from other forms of dementia. Because an ApoE4 test can only suggest probabilities, not predict or rule out AD with certainty, its usefulness in the absence of proven treatments is dubious. Dr. Rudolph E. Tanzi feels the test, if positive, is more likely to produce stress and anxiety than productive results.[30]

While the ApoE4 gene may be stacked against us, some of our most senior citizens could harbor genetic defenses against AD. Surprisingly, people living to the age of 100 and beyond seem to flip AD probabilities upside down. They are rarely affected, which flies in the face of overwhelming evidence that the incidence of the disease increases with age. This paradox has fueled detailed investigations into what role genes might play in bequeathing "AD immunity" to the few of us who make it into a second century.[31]

Quite obviously, we have a lot to learn about the genetics behind Alzheimer's, but the Human Genome Project, to be discussed shortly, should help minimize our confusion.

Making this cycle even more vicious is another unfortunate fact of life in the Alzheimer's brain, Dr. Li says. For reasons not yet fully understood, the blood vessels of people with AD appear to give off a toxin that kills brain cells directly. "In a way, it's as though the blood vessels are an ambulance crew that shows up, only to begin harming the very people they were sent to help," Dr. Li says.

But why would the body want to play such a cruel trick on itself? "That's the big question we're still trying to answer," Dr. Li says. "Probably there are a variety of influences including genetics, environment, and lifestyle factors. Alzheimer's is an extremely complicated disease that we're just beginning to understand."

As the Angiogenesis Foundation is searching for the "why" of Alzheimer's disease, it's also looking for the "what to do about it," and it hopes to break new ground here, too. Researchers have known for years that people who take medicines like nonsteroidal anti-inflammatory drugs have a much lower risk of Alzheimer's, and efforts are under way to understand how brain inflammation makes Alzheimer's disease worse. "We've taken this observation in a new direction, because many anti-inflammatory drugs inhibit angiogenesis," says Dr. Li. "We think that antiangiogenesis medicines may help prevent Alzheimer's by stopping the growth of those damaging blood vessel cells."

> *Researchers have known for years that people who take medicines like nonsteroidal anti-inflammatory drugs have a much lower risk of Alzheimer's, and efforts are under way to understand how brain inflammation makes Alzheimer's disease worse.*

The Angiogenesis Foundation is now conducting research into other medicines that suppress angiogenesis, some now used for cancer and other diseases, and that may have the potential for preventing Alzheimer's. "There's now an explosion of new discoveries in medical research," says Dr. Li. "It's going to become increasingly more important for different fields of scientific endeavor to communicate about what they're learning. Only through this kind of cross-pollination of knowledge will real progress be able to flower."

More than 60 drugs currently are being developed to stop angiogenesis associated with cancer, for example, and with the right kind of scientific sharing, Dr. Li says, some of these could have important uses in treating Alzheimer's disease, too. "Anti-inflammatory drugs such as the COX-2 inhibitors used for treating arthritis, and drugs to treat high cholesterol and high blood pressure, also are showing promise as angiogenesis inhibitors, so we're excited about the potential of these in the fight against Alzheimer's as well," he says.

Even contributions from Mother Nature are showing promise. Soy protein and green tea are natural sources of angiogenesis inhibitors. "We need to open our eyes to all the possibilities," Dr. Li says. "And when we do, it's my guess we'll be finding ways to beat not just Alzheimer's but a lot of other diseases as well."

For more information on angiogenesis or research being done by the Angiogenesis Foundation, check its Web site at www.angio.org.

SERENDIPITY

Somewhat surprisingly, many medications used in the treatment of ulcers, high blood pressure, headaches, and other common ailments seem to ward off Alzheimer's disease. Let's learn about a few of them and their possible role in treating AD.

> *More than 60 drugs currently are being developed to stop angiogenesis associated with cancer, for example, and with the right kind of scientific sharing, Dr. Li says, some of these could have important uses in treating Alzheimer's disease, too.*

Ibuprofen

Some evidence indicates that ibuprofen, an anti-inflammatory drug, has a slight protective effect when taken in normal doses, which scientists attribute to a moderation of brain inflammation linked with Alzheimer's. However, in large doses given to mice, the drug had a completely different effect, according to a recent study in *Nature*. It blocked production of amyloid-beta 42, the protein responsible for plaque formation in people with Alzheimer's.[32] Before renting a pickup truck for a trip to the drugstore, however, it's important to note that the large doses used in the study would cause serious gastrointestinal and kidney problems in humans. "If people go out and start taking buckets of Advil, we'd be in big trouble," reported University of California–San Diego researcher Edward Koo.[33] First, we must solve the toxicity problem.

Clioquinol

Another candidate for treatment of AD is a 1950's antibiotic, clioquinol. The drug was pulled off the market when suspected of causing neurological problems and then later cleared for human use. During initial tests with transgenic mice, clioquinol dissolved plaque and improved mental function.

Unlike other plaque inhibitors, clioquinol targets harmful metals, specifically copper and zinc, which occur at unusually high levels in the brains of people with Alzheimer's. According to the theory behind this approach, these metals not only combine with normal proteins in the brain to form neuron-destroying plaque but also produce free radicals that kill healthy cells. "Cataracts, Lou Gehrig's disease, spongiform encephalopathies, and Parkinson's disease—these have in common a protein that binds a metal that we think is responsible for spawning free radicals," said Ashley I. Bush, M.D., Ph.D., director of the laboratory for oxidation biology at Harvard University. "This is potentially a change in understanding Alzheimer's disease and other degenerative disorders where there is a metal involved," Dr. Bush explained. "We think this could be a whole new class of therapeutic agent. We are very optimistic about the possibilities."[34]

> *Unlike other plaque inhibitors, clioquinol targets harmful metals, specifically copper and zinc, which occur at unusually high levels in the brains of people with Alzheimer's.*

As of June 2001, human studies with clioquinol were under way in Australia, and the drug had proved safe when taken in combination with vitamin B_{12} supplements.[35]

Statins

Already known to be safe are statins, commonly recognized as Lipitor, Zocor, and Pravachol, because they are used daily throughout the world to lower cholesterol, thereby reducing heart attacks and strokes. Recent findings suggest statins fend off mental decline as well. "What we found," said Dr. Benjamin Wolozin of Loyola University Medical Center outside Chicago, "was that patients taking statins have a 60 to 70 percent reduction in the risk of Alzheimer's disease." Even doubters were impressed when a second study conducted by a different research group came to the same conclusion.[36]

Evidence from animal studies in which cholesterol has been linked to the accumulation of plaque in the brain explains why statins may mitigate the risks of mental decline. Studies are being conducted in the United States and Europe to further clarify the connection between cholesterol and brain function as well as to determine what future role statins might play in the war against AD.[37]

Solving the Mystery

So where do all these seemingly haphazard connections leave us? "With very important clues," answers Dr. Li. "Alzheimer's is a complex disease probably triggered by a variety of mechanisms. The faster we uncover new clues and piece them together, the sooner we will unravel its mysteries."

> *E*vidence from animal studies in which cholesterol has been linked to the accumulation of plaque in the brain explains why statins may mitigate the risks of mental decline.

BETTER DIAGNOSTIC TECHNIQUES

Alzheimer's disease is not easily identified. Consequently, as new treatments come along, we will have to sharpen our diagnostic capabilities to prescribe the best course of therapy.

When a person has trouble with recollection or other mental activities, the clinician typically employs tests of memory, verbal skills, and other mental functions, as well as an evaluation of behavior, to make a diagnosis of "possible" or "probable" AD. Before placing a person in the "probable" category, efforts are normally made to rule out other potential causes, such as substance abuse, Parkinson's disease, stroke, or tumor. Eliminating the latter two possibilities may require a brain scan.[38]

Also, Parkinson's disease may be impossible to exclude due to a growing body of evidence demonstrating common physical symptoms and neuroanatomy.[39] For instance, some people with AD exhibit the same problems with movement as do people with Parkinson's disease. During autopsy, both diseases often display identical characteristics, including changes in the substantia nigra (an area controlling movement) and the presence of Lewy bodies (neuron pathology markers), as well as the plaques and neurofibrillary tangles associated with AD. In fact, human brains showing signs of both diseases are common.[40]

As a result, some clinicians propose that Alzheimer's and Parkinson's are the same disease occurring under the broader umbrella of a single neurological pathology. A counterargument contends that one person can have both diseases at the same time and that many people often do.[41]

> Some clinicians propose that Alzheimer's and Parkinson's are the same disease occurring under the broader umbrella of a single neurological pathology.

What should be clear is that diagnosing AD is not an exact science, even in the coroner's office. Nevertheless, the earlier the disease is detected, the more effectively symptoms can be managed. With the development of effective treatments on the horizon, an early, accurate diagnosis of Alzheimer's could mean the difference between a retirement sprinkled with happy days on the golf course and one filled with suffering.

Detecting Mild Cognitive Impairment

A major area of focus for researchers in pursuit of better diagnostic techniques is on people with mild cognitive impairment. Generally speaking, these people decline mentally more quickly than their peers, but they remain outside the clinical parameters defining AD. Why are these people of such interest? Because approximately 40 percent of them will develop the disease within 3 years, while others with mild cognitive impairment will never suffer from AD. The challenge for researchers is to identify warning signs that put individuals within this group most at risk. By doing so, they will be better able to assist clinicians in getting a head start on diagnosis and treatment.[42]

Brain Imaging

Another tool with the potential for playing a critical role in early diagnosis of AD is brain imaging. With magnetic resonance imaging (MRI), researchers can now measure different regions within the brain, including the hippocampus, which begins to decrease in size during the earliest stages of the disease. Two other imaging technologies, positron emission tomography (PET) and single photon emission computer tomography (SPECT), display actual brain activity, which can then be cross-referenced with what the person is doing at the time. In this way, researchers are able to map those areas of the brain used for reading, talking, recalling, and performing other mental operations. It's hoped that these "live-action" scanning techniques will provide today's researchers and tomorrow's clinicians with a powerful tool for detecting AD in its earliest stages.[43]

How the Human Genome Project Will Help

Quite frankly, these evolving tools pale when compared to the nearly omniscient diagnostic magic that may be available in less than a decade. The "sorcery" will spring from the Human Genome Project, whose goals are to identify all the genes (approximately 30,000) in human DNA; determine the sequences of the 3 billion base pairs making up human DNA; store this information in databases; improve tools for analyzing genetic data; transfer related technologies to the private sector; and address the ethical, legal, and social issues arising from the project.[44]

In simpler terms, the Human Genome Project focuses on the architects who design our bodies, the genes carrying all the information needed to assemble the proteins from which we are made. When genes are defective, so are we, to greater and lesser degrees. Down's syndrome, a specific type of "at-conception" mental retardation also identifiable by physical abnormalities, offers an example of an architect gone awry. Like a number of other human afflictions, Down's syndrome can be linked to a single chromosome, an architect who passed on the wrong blueprints. However, the genetic culprits in most human afflictions, particularly those associated with aging, aren't so easy to pick out in a chromosomal "lineup." Typically, they commit crimes against our bodies in gangs whose members change from one assault (for example, cancer, heart disease, arthritis, Alzheimer's) to the next.

The Human Genome Project focuses on the architects who design our bodies, the genes carrying all the information needed to assemble the proteins from which we are made.

Through the Human Genome Project, expected to be completed in 2003, we will go far beyond rounding up the "usual suspects." As our mug file (a computer-based cross-reference between genetic patterns and disease expression) grows, we will pick up the perpetrators before the crime is even committed. In other words, we will anticipate assaults on our health and take the appropriate defensive measures before the propensity for a disease manifests itself as the actual disease. A continually expanding medical file on the human race will enable us to refine our defenses so they protect us where we are most vulnerable without compromising our strengths. In short, we will benefit from increasingly effective treatments with progressively fewer undesirable side effects.

RESEARCH UPDATES

As mentioned earlier in this chapter, secrecy surrounds many of the efforts being aimed at the development of new Alzheimer's treatments. Staying abreast of the progress being made against AD can be difficult, therefore, but a nonprofit organization known as the Alzeimer Research Forum has recognized this information gap and sought to bridge it via its Web site at www.alzforum.org. Intended for scientists and the general public alike, the site provides updates on the latest advances in research, gives information on the availability of support groups and clinical trials for new drugs, offers on-line

Early Birds and Ulcers

Although the early bird may get the worm, it could also end up with an ulcer, or even more serious complications, by trying to fend off Alzheimer's with unproven and unapproved treatments. Just because many nonsteroidal anti-inflammatory drugs, such as ibuprofen, are available without a prescription does not mean we can take them without risk. All ibuprofen products (Advil, Motrin, Nuprin) can cause major gastrointestinal problems. More important, they may not work in preventing or slowing the onset of Alzheimer's, which explains why they are still in clinical trials and not yet approved by the FDA for treatment of the disease. In a nutshell, there is no compelling evidence to date that ibuprofen's benefits outweigh its risks in the context of AD.

Putting aside the complex subject of contraindications (mismatches of drugs with a person's medical profile or other drugs being taken), let's note some of the adverse effects of drugs now being evaluated for Alzheimer's treatment. They include liver damage, upper respiratory tract infection, diarrhea, nausea, heartburn, higher blood pressure, swelling of the lower legs and feet, and more intense body odor.

Our recommendation: Be an early bird by keeping your eyes and ears open concerning developments in the war against Alzheimer's, but beware of "good news" not supported by reputable studies, your physician, and the FDA. You want *the* worm, not a can full of them.

discussion forums, and even provides news updates via e-mail on a weekly basis. It's a "must-see" for anyone interested in staying on top of the latest developments in this ever-advancing field of medical research.

THE CURE: WHAT, WHEN, AND HOW?

For the better part of this decade, we will probably conduct a defensive war, highlighted by major treatment successes, against Alzheimer's. These efforts will most likely include multiple tactics, such as improved screening to detect people most at risk, compounds to inhibit the formation and aggregation of beta-amyloid, anti-inflammatory drugs to reduce swelling, antioxidants to reduce cell stress, cholinesterase drugs to combat chemical deficiencies, and neuroprotectants and/or regenerators to bolster the population of neuronal cells. Because the most common type of Alzheimer's occurs in old age, slowing its onset by 5 or 10 years could reduce its incidence by 50 to 75 percent.[45] In terms of reduced human suffering, these first small steps would represent a major leap forward, indeed.

But looking ahead a bit further (perhaps into the next decade), these hunt-and-peck approaches should appear crude to us in retrospect as the Human Genome Project explodes with information to fuel precision therapies. Paul Raia, Ph.D., director of patient care and family support at the Alzheimer's Association of Eastern Massachusetts, sums up hope for the future with a negative slant. "I'll be out of a job in 7 to 10 years," he predicts.

That's great news for all of us—including Dr. Raia, too, no doubt.

Appendix: Resources

NATIONAL ORGANIZATIONS

Administration on Aging
330 Independence Avenue, S.W.
Washington, DC 20201
Phone: (202) 619-7501
Web site: www.aoa.dhhs.gov

**Alliance for Children
and Families**
11700 West Lake Park Drive
Milwaukee, WI 53224
Phone: (414) 359-1040
Web site: www.alliance1.org

The Alzheimer's Association
919 North Michigan Avenue,
    Suite 1100
Chicago, IL 60611
Phone: (800) 272-3900
Web site: www.alz.org

**American Association of
Retired Persons**
601 E Street, N.W.
Washington, DC 20049
Phone: (800) 424-3410

Web site: www.aarp.org
(Ask for caregiver resource kit D15267.)

American Geriatrics Society
350 Fifth Avenue, Suite 801
New York, NY 10118
Phone: (212) 308-1414
Web site: www.americangeriatrics
    .org

American Society on Aging
833 Market Street, Suite 512
San Francisco, CA 94103
Phone: (415) 974-9600
Web site: www.asaging.org

Family Caregiver Alliance
690 Market Street, Suite 600
San Francisco, CA 94104
Phone: (415) 434-3388
Web site: www.caregiver.org

Interfaith Caregivers Alliance
112 West 9th, Suite 600
Kansas City, MO 64105

Phone: (816) 913-5442
Web site: www.interfaithcaregivers
    .org

**The National Family Caregiver's
Association (NFCA)**
10400 Connecticut Avenue,
    Suite 500
Kensington, MD 20895
Phone: (800) 896-3650
Web site: www.nfcacares.org

**National Institute of
Mental Health**
6001 Executive Boulevard
Room 8184, MSC 9663
Bethesda, MD 20892

Phone: (301) 443-4513
Web site: www-srb.nimh.nih.gov
    /gi.html

National Institute on Aging
31 Center Drive
Building 31, Room 5C27, MSC 2292
Bethesda, MD 20892
Phone: (301) 496-1752
Web site: www.nia.nih.gov

**Visiting Nurse Associations
of America**
11 Beacon Street, Suite 910
Boston, MA 02108
Phone: (888) 866-8773
Web site: www.vnaa.org

CARE-FACILITY ORGANIZATIONS

**American Association of Homes
and Services for the Aging**
2519 Connecticut Avenue, N.W.
Washington, DC 20008
Phone: (202) 738-2241
Web site: www.aahsa.org

**American Health Care
Association**
1201 L Street, N.W.
Washington, DC 20005
Phone: (202) 842-4444
Web site: www.ahca.org

**Assisted Living Federation
of America**
11200 Waples Mill Road, Suite 150
Fairfax, VA 22030

Phone: (703) 691-8100
Web site: www.alfa.org

Eldercare Locator
Phone: (800) 677-1116
Web site: www.eldercare.gov

**The National Council on
the Aging**
409 Third Street, S.W.,
    Suite 200
Washington, DC 20024
Phone: (202) 479-1200
Web site: www.ncoa.org

Senior Alternatives
Web site: www.senioralternatives
    .com

ORGANIZATIONS TO ASSIST WITH LEGAL AND FINANICAL ISSUES

The Financial Planning Association
Phone: (800) 282-7526
Web site: www.fpanet.org/planner
    search

National Academy of Elder Law Attorneys, Inc.
Phone: (520) 881-4005
Web site: www.naela.org

National Senior Citizens Law Center
Washington, DC, office
    Phone: (202) 289-6976
Los Angeles, CA, office
    Phone: (213) 639-0930
Oakland, CA, office
    Phone: (510) 663-1132
Web site: www.nsclc.org

INTERNET RESOURCES

The Alzheimer's Disease Education and Referral Center (ADEAR)
Web site: www.alzheimers.org

Alzheimer's Disease International
Web site: www.alz.co.uk

Alzheimer Research Forum
Web site: www.alzforum.org

Alzheimer Society of Canada
Web site: www.alzheimer.ca

Alzheimer Web
Web site: http://werple.mira.net.au
    /~dhs/ad.html

American Journal of Alzheimer's Disease and Other Dementias
Web site: www.alzheimersjournal
    .com/pn02000.html

CareGuide.com
Web site: www.careguide.com

Doctor's Guide
Web site: www.pslgroup.com
    /alzheimer.htm

Mental Health InfoSource
Web site: www.mhsource.com
    /disorders/dementia.html

Resources for Enhancing Alzheimer's Caregiver Health (REACH)
Web site: www.edc.gsph.pitt.edu
    /reach/info.html

Volunteers of America
Web site: www.voa.org

ONLINE DISCUSSION GROUPS

Alzheimer's Discussion Group
Web site: http://sargon.mmu.ac.uk
  /alzhimer.htm

Caregiving.com
Web site: www.caregiving.com

Alzheimer's Webforum
Web site: http://neuro-www.mgh
  .harvard.edu/forum/Alzheimers
  DiseaseMenu.html

SUPPORT GROUPS

The Alzheimer's Association
Phone: (800) 272-3900
Web site: www.alz.org

**Friends and Relatives of
Institutionalized Aged**
Phone: (212) 732-4455
Web site: www.fria.org

**Alzheimer's Disease Education
and Referral Center (ADEAR)**
Phone: (800) 438-4380
Web site: www.alzheimers.org

**National Association
of Home Care**
Phone: (202) 547-7424
Web site: www.nahc.org

Children of Aging Parents
Phone: (800) 227-7294
Web site: www.caps4caregivers
  .org

Well Spouse Foundation
Phone: (800) 838-0879
Web site: www.wellspouse.org

NEWSLETTERS AND MAGAZINES

The Caregiver Newsletter
Duke Family Support Program
Duke University Medical Center
P.O. Box 3600
Durham, NC 27710
Phone: (919) 660-7510

Today's Caregiver Magazine
6365 Taft Street,
  Suite 3006
Hollywood, FL 33024
Phone: (800) 829-2734
Web site: www.caregiver.com

RECOMMENDED READING

Aging with Grace: What the Nun Study Teaches Us About Leading Longer, Healthier, and More Meaningful Lives by David Snowdon, Ph.D. (Bantam, 2001).

Alzheimer's Early Stages: First Steps in Caring and Treatment by Daniel Kuhn, M.S.W. (Hunter House, 1999).

Alzheimer's Disease: Frequently Asked Questions by Frena Gray-Davidson (McGraw-Hill, 1999).

Decoding Darkness: The Search for the Genetic Causes of Alzheimer's Disease by Rudolph E. Tanzi and Anne B. Parsons (Perseus, 2001).

The Forgetting: Alzheimer's: Portrait of an Epidemic by David Shenk (Doubleday, 2001).

Speaking Our Minds: Personal Reflections from Individuals with Alzheimer's by Lisa Snyder, L.C.S.W. (Freeman, 2000).

Your Name Is Hughes Hannibal Shanks: A Caregiver's Guide to Alzheimer's by Lela Knox Shanks (Penguin, 1999).

What You Need to Know About Alzheimer's Disease by John J. Medina, Ph.D. (New Harbinger, 1999).

Notes

Introduction

1. Alzheimer's Association, *Alzheimer's Disease Caregiver's Survey* (Chicago: Alzheimer's Association, 1996), 3.
2. A.T. Hingley, *Alzheimer's: Few Clues on the Mystery of Memory*, U.S. Food and Drug Administration, www.fda.gov/fdac/features/1998/398_alz.html, accessed Sept. 8, 2001.
3. Ibid.
4. "Caregiver and Clinician Communication," *Harvard Women's Health Watch* viii, no. 12 (August 2001): 6.
5. Ibid.

Chapter 1

1. D. Kuhn, *Alzheimer's Early Stages* (Alameda, CA: Hunter House, 1999): 13
2. J. Medina, *What You Need to Know About Alzheimer's Disease* (Hong Kong: CME and New Harbinger, 1999): 11.
3. Ibid., 12.
4. Kuhn, *Alzheimer's Early Stages*: 8.
5. National Institute on Aging and National Institutes of Health, *2000 Progress Report on Alzheimer's Disease*, NIH Publication no. 00-4859 (Washington, D.C.: Government Printing Office, 2000).
6. Ibid.
7. K. Garber, "An End to Alzheimer's ?" *Technology Review: MIT's Magazine of Innovation* 104, no. 2 (March, 2001).
8. "General Statistics/Demographics," Alzheimer's Association, www.alz .org/hc/overview/stats/htm, accessed September 29, 2001.
9. L. Snyder, *Speaking Our Minds* (New York: Freeman, 1999): 6.

10. Medina, *What You Need to Know About Alzheimer's Disease*.

11. "General Statistics/Demographics," Alzheimer's Association, www.alz.org /hc/overview/stats/htm, accessed September 29, 2002.

12. Snyder, *Speaking Our Minds*: 17.

13. Kuhn, *Alzheimer's Early Stages:* 29; see also "Alzheimer's Disease," Mayo Clinic.com., www.mayoclinic.com.

14. Kuhn, *Alzheimer's Early Stages:* 27.

15. Ibid., 27.

16. Medina, *What You Need to Know About Alzheimer's Disease*.

17. Kuhn, *Alzheimer's Early Stages:* 27.

18. National Institute on Aging and National Institutes of Health, *2000 Progress Report on Alzheimer's Disease*.

19. "General Statistics/Demographics," Alzheimer's Association, www.alz.org /research/current/statistics.htm, accessed September 29, 2001.

20. J.C. Breitner, "Family Aggregation in Alzheimer's Disease: Comparison of Risk Among Relatives of Early- and Late-Onset Cases, and Among Male and Female Relatives in Successive Generations," *Neurology* 38 (1988): 207–212.

21. P.N. Nemetz, "Traumatic Head Injury and Time of Onset to Alzheimer's Disease: A Population Study," *American Journal of Epidemiology* 149 (1999): 32–40.

22. D.A. Evans, "Education and Other Measures of Socioeconomic Status and Risk of Incident Alzheimer's Disease in a Defined Population of Older Persons," *Archives of Neurology* 54, no. 11 (1997): 1399–1405.

23. K.E. Wisniewski, "Occurrence of Neuropathological Changes and Dementia of Alzheimer's Disease in Down's Syndrome," *Annals of Neurology* 17 (1985): 278–282.

24. H. Payami, "Increased Risk of Familial Late-Onset Alzheimer's Disease in Women," *Neurology* 46 (1996): 126–129; L. Letenneur, "Are Sex and Educational Level Independent Risk Factors of Dementia and Alzheimer's Disease?" *Journal of Neurology, Neurosurgery and Psychiatry* 66 (1999): 177–183.

25. D.A. Snowden, "Brain Infarction and Clinical Expression of Alzheimer's Disease: The Nun Study," *Journal of the American Medical Association* 277, no. 10 (1997): 813–817.

26. R.A. Armstrong, "Aluminum and Alzheimer's Disease: Review of Possible Pathogenic Mechanisms," *Dementia* 7, no. 1 (1996): 1–9.

27. W.R. Markesbury, "Trace Elements in Alzheimer's Disease," in *Alzheimer's Disease: Causes, Diagnosis, Treatment and Care*, ed. Z. S. Khacha-

turian and T.S. Radebaugh (Boca Raton, FL: CRC, 1996), 233–236; and S.R. Saxe, "Alzheimer's Disease, Dental Amalgam and Mercury," *Journal of the American Dental Association* 130 (1999): 191–199.

28. W.A. Kukall, "Solvent Exposure As a Risk Factor for Alzheimer's Disease: A Case-Control Study," *American Journal of Epidemiology* 141, no. 11 (1995): 1059–1071.

29. Canadian Study of Health and Aging Investigators, "The Canadian Study of Health and Aging: Risk Factors for Alzheimer's Disease in Canada," *Neurology* 40 (1994): 1492–1495.

30. A. Ott, "Smoking and the Risk of Dementia and Alzheimer's Disease in a Population-Based Cohort Study: The Rotterdam Study," *The Lancet* 351, no. 9119 (1998) 1840–1843.

31. C. Merchant, "The Influence of Smoking on the Risk of Alzheimer's Disease," *Neurology* 52, no. 7 (1999): 1408–1412.

32. National Institute on Aging and National Institutes of Health, *2000 Progress Report on Alzheimer's Disease*.

33. S. Kalmijn, "Polyunsaturated Fatty Foods, Antioxidants and Cognitive Function in the Very Old," *American Journal of Epidemiology* 145 (1994): 33–41.

34. R. Clarke, "Folate, Vitamin B_{12} and Serum Total Homocysteine Levels in Confirmed Alzheimer's Disease," *Archives of Neurology* 55 (1998): 1449–1455.

35. A.L. Smith, "The Protective Effects of Life-Long, Regular Physical Exercise on the Development of Alzheimer's Disease," *Neurology* 50, no. 4, suppl. (1998), a presentation at the Fiftieth Annual Meeting of the American Academy of Neurology, Minneapolis, MN, April 29, 1998.

36. National Institute on Aging and National Institutes of Health, *2000 Progress Report on Alzheimer's Disease*.

37. J.S. Kennedy, "Alzheimer's Disease," *Clinical Geriatric Neurology*, ed. L. Barclay (Malvern, PA: Lea & Febinger, 1993): 76–89.

38. M.X. Tang, "The APOE-E4 Allele and the Risk of Alzheimer's Disease Among African Americans, Whites and Hispanics," *Journal of the American Medical Association* 279, no. 10 (1998): 751–755.

39. R.N. Rosenberg, "Genetic Factors for the Development of Alzheimer's Disease in the Cherokee Indian," *Archives of Neurology* 53, no. 10 (1996): 997–1000.

40. L. White, "Prevalence of Dementia in Older Japanese-American Men in Hawaii," *Journal of the American Medical Association* 276, no. 12 (1996): 955–960.

Chapter 2

1. D. Shenk, *The Forgetting—Alzheimer's: Portrait of an Epidemic* (New York: Doubleday, 2001): 34.
2. F. Gray-Davidson, *Alzheimer's Disease: Frequently Asked Questions* (Los Angeles, CA: McGraw Hill, 1999): 23.
3. Ibid., 25.
4. Ibid.
5. L. Snyder, *Speaking Our Minds* (New York: Freeman, 2000): 6.
6. A.T. Hingley, "Alzheimer's: Few Clues on the Mysteries of Memory," U.S. Food and Drug Administration, www.fda.gov/fdac/features/1998/398_alz.html, accessed September 1, 2001.
7. D.P. Devanand et al., "Olfactory Deficits in Patients with Mild Cognitive Impairment Predict Alzheimer's Disease at Follow-Up," *American Journal of Psychiatry*, 157 (September 2000): 1399–1405.
8. Gray-Davidson, *Alzheimer's Disease:* 25.
9. J.C. Mundt, "Computer-Automated Dementia Screening Using a Touch-Tone Telephone," *Archives of Internal Medicine* 161 (2001): 2481–2487.
10. Folstein, et al., "Mini Mental State," *Journal of Psychiatric Research* 12: 196–198 (1975).
11. National Institute on Aging and the National Institutes of Health, *2000 Progress Report on Alzheimer's Disease*, NIH publication no. 00–4859 (Washington, D.C.: Government Printing Office, 2000): 12.
12. "Caregiver and Clinician Communication," *Harvard Women's Health Watch* viii, no. 12 (August 2000): 6.
13. D. Kuhn, *Alzheimer's Early Stages* (Alameda, CA: Hunter House, 1999): 21.
14. Shenk, *The Forgetting:* 115.
15. Kuhn, *Alzheimer's Early Stages:* 18.
16. B. Reisberg, "Retrogenesis: Clinical, Physiologic, and Pathologic Mechanisms in Brain Aging, Alzheimer's and Other Dementing Processes," *European Archive of Psychiatry in Clinical Neurosciences* 249, suppl. 3 (1999).

Chapter 3

1. S.L. Rogers, L.T. Friedhoff, and the Donepezil Study Group, "The Efficacy and Safety of Donepezil in Patients with Alzheimer's Disease: Results of a U.S. Multicentre, Randomized, Double-Blind, Placebo-Controlled Trial," *Dementia* 7, no. 6 (1996): 293–303; and R. Anand and G. Gharabawi, "Efficacy and Safety Results of the Early Phases with Exelon (ENA 713) in Alzheimer's Disease: An Overview," *Journal of Drug Development in Clinical Practice* 8 (1996): 109–116.

2. D. Kuhn, *Alzheimer's Early Stages:* 64.

3. D. Snowdon, *Aging with Grace* (New York: Bantam, 2001): 123.

4. Rogers et al., "The Efficacy and Safety of Donepezil."

5. M. Rosler et al., "Efficacy and Safety of Rivastigimine in Patients with Alzheimer's Disease: International Randomised Controlled Trial," *British Medical Journal* 18 (1999): 633–640.

6. J. Coyle, "Galantamine, a Cholinesterase Inhibitor That Allosterically Modulates Nicotinic Receptors: Effects on the Course of Alzheimer's Disease," *Biological Psychiatry*, 49 (February 2001): 289–299.

7. Kuhn, *Alzheimer's Early Stages:* 74.

8. Ibid., 75.

9. J.A. Duke, *The Green Pharmacy* (New York: St. Martin's, 1998): 46.

10. Kuhn, *Alzheimer's Early Stages:* 76.

11. S.S. Xu et al., "Efficacy of Tablet Huperzine-A on Memory, Cognition and Behavior in Alzheimer's Disease," *Zhongguo Yao Li Xue Bao* 16 (1995): 391–395.

12. Q.Q. Sun et al., "Huperzine-A Capsules Enhance Memory and Learning Performance in 34 Pairs of Matched Adolescent Students," *Zhongguo Yao Li Xue Bao* 20 (1999): 601–603.

13. P.L. LeBars, M.M. Katz, N. Berman, et al., "A Placebo-Controlled Double-Blind, Randomized Trial of an Extract of Gingko Biloba for Dementia," North American EGb Study Group, *Journal of the American Medical Association* 278 (1997): 1327–1332.

14. J.A. Mix and W.D. Crews, Jr., "An Examination of the Efficacy of Gingko Biloba Extract EGb 761 on the Neuropsychologic Functioning of Cognitively Intact Older Adults," *Journal of Complimentary Medicine* 6 (2000): 219–229.

15. I. Hindmarch, "Activity of Gingko Biloba Extract on Short-Term Memory" [in French with an English abstract], *Presse Med* 5 (1986): 1592–1594.

16. S. Bratman, "Alzheimer's Disease, Non-Alzheimer's Dementia, and Normal Age-Related Memory Loss," The Natural Pharmacist (TNP .com), www.tnp.com/encyclopedia/condition/151/17/, accessed August 16, 2001.

17. T. Cenacchi, T. Bertoldin, C. Farina, et al., "Cognitive Decline in the Elderly: A Double-Blind, Placebo-Controlled Multicenter Study on Efficacy of Phosphatidylserine Administration," *Aging* (Milan) 5 (1993): 123–133.

18. P.J. Delwaide, A.M. Gyselynck-Mambourg, A. Hurlet, et al., "Double-Blind, Randomized Controlled Study of Phosphatidylserine in Senile

Demented Patients," *Acta Neurologica Scandinavica* 73 (1986): 136–140; and T.H. Crook, J. Tinklenberg, J. Yesavage, et al., "Effects of Phosphatidylserine on Age-Related Memory Impairment," *Neurology* 41 (1991): 644–649.

19. P.C. Bickford et al., "Antioxidant-Rich Diets Improve Cerebellar Physiology and Motor Learning in Aged Rats," *Brain Research* 866, nos. 1–2 (2000): 211–217.

20. "What Are the Latest Drug Treatments for Alzheimer's Disease?" CBS Healthwatch, http://cbshealthwatch.medscape.com/cx/viewarticle/401936, accessed September 19, 2001.

21. L. Teri et al., "Treatment of Agitation in AD: A Randomized, Placebo-Controlled Clinical Trial," *Neurology* 9 (2000): 1271–1278.

22. "Treating Agitation (Behavioral Symptoms)," Alzheimer's Association, www.alz.org/caregiver/undertstanding/treatment/behavioral.htm; and "Treating Behavioral Symptoms," Alzheimer's Association, www.alz.org/hc/treatments/behaviors/htm, accessed October 30, 2001.

23. P.L. McGeer, M. Schulzer, and E.G. McGeer, "Arthritis and Anti-inflammatory Agents as Possible Protective Factors Against Alzheimer's Disease: A Review of 17 Epidemiological Studies," *Neurology* 47 (1996): 425–432.

24. J.B. Rich et al., "Nonsteroidal Anti-Inflammatory Drugs in Alzheimer's Disease," *Neurology* 46 (1995): 626–632.

25. G.R. Lim et al., "Ibuprofen Suppresses Plaque Pathology and Inflammation in a Mouse Model for Alzheimer's Disease," *Journal of Neuroscience* 20 (2000): 5709–5714.

26. Snowdon, *Aging with Grace:* 181.

27. M.X. Tang et al., "Effect of Estrogen During Menopause on Risk and Age of Onset of Alzheimer's Disease," *The Lancet* 248 (1996): 429–432; and C. Kawas et al., "A Prospective Study of Estrogen Replacement Therapy and the Risk of Developing Alzheimer's Disease; The Baltimore Longitudinal Study of Aging," *Neurology* 48, no. 6 (1997): 1517–1521.

28. R.A. Mulnard et al., "Estrogen Replacement Therapy for the Treatment of Mild to Moderate Alzheimer's Disease: A Randomized Controlled Trial. Alzheimer's Disease Cooperative Study," *Journal of the American Medical Association* 283, no. 8 (2000): 1007–1015; and V.W. Henderson, et al., "Estrogen for Alzheimer's Disease in Women: Randomized, Double-Blind, Placebo-Controlled Trial," *Neurology* 54, no. 2 (2000): 295–301.

29. M. Sano et al., "A Controlled Trial of Selegiline, Alpha-Tocopherol or Both as Treatment for Alzheimer's Disease," *New England Journal of Medicine* 336 (1997): 1216–1222.

30. National Institute on Aging and National Institutes of Health, *2000 Progress Report on Alzheimer's Disease*, NIH Publication no. 00-4859 (Washington, D.C.: Government Printing Office, 2000): 36.

31. D. Shenk, *The Forgetting—Alzheimer's: Portrait of an Epidemic* (New York: Doubleday, 2001): 203.

32. C.H. Espinel, "De Kooning's Late Colours and Forms: Dementia, Creativity, and the Healing Power of Art," *The Lancet* 20 (April 1996).

33. K. Larson, "Alzheimer's Expressionism," *Village Voice* (May 31, 1994).

34. F. Gray-Davidson, *Alzheimer's Disease: Frequently Asked Questions* (Los Angeles: Lowell House, 1999): 151.

35. Ibid.

Chapter 4

1. D. Kuhn, *Alzheimer's Early Stages* (Alameda, CA: Hunter House, 1999): 80.

2. J. Medina, *What You Need to Know About Alzheimer's Disease* (Hong Kong: CME and New Harbinger, 1999): 110.

3. Kuhn, *Alzheimer's Early Stages*: 21.

4. Ibid., 85.

5. J.C. Rogers, "Improving Morning Care Routines of Nursing Home Residents with Dementia," *Journal of the American Geriatrics Society* 47 (1999): 1049–1057.

6. Medina, *What You Need to Know About Alzheimer's Disease:* 110.

7. F. Gray-Davidson, *Alzheimer's Disease: Frequently Asked Questions* (Los Angeles: Lowell House, 1999): 151.

8. Medina, *What You Need to Know About Alzheimer's Disease:* 127.

9. D.B. Carr, "Motor Vehicle Crashes and Drivers with DAT," *Alzheimer's Disease and Associated Disorders* 11, suppl. 1 (1997): 38–41.

10. N.L. Mace and P.V. Rabins, *The 36-Hour Day* (New York: Warner, 1999): 321.

11. M.A. Wilson, "Fit at Fifty . . . and Beyond," Mature Fitness, www.seniorfitness.net/fitfifty.htm, accessed September 26, 2001.

12. P.J. Bird, "Exercise and Alzheimer's Disease," University of Florida College of Health and Human Performance, www.hhp.ufl.edu/keepingfit/article/exalz.htm, accessed November 4, 2001.

13. M.E. Nelson and S. Wernick, *Strong Women Stay Young* (New York: Bantam, 1997): 74.

14. R. Garnett, *The Life of Ralph Waldo Emerson* (New York: Haskell House, [1888] 1974): 211.

15. C. Henderson and R.D. Henderson, *Partial View: An Alzheimer's Journal* (Dallas: Southern Methodist University, 1998): 55.

16. L. Rose, *Show Me the Way Home* (Forest Knolls, CA: Elder Books, 1996): 35.

17. C. Boden, *Who Will I Be When I Die?* (East Melbourne, Australia: HarperCollins Religious, 1998): 53.

18. K. Langa, "National Estimates of the Quality and Cost of Informal Caregiving for the Elderly with Dementia," *Journal of General Internal Medicine*, (November 16, 2001): 770–778.

Chapter 5

1. Alzheimer's Association, *Alzheimer's Disease Caregiver's Survey* (Chicago: Alzheimer's Association, 1996): 3.

2. T. Hamazaki et al., "The Effect of Docosahexaenic Acid on Aggression in Young Adults," *Journal of Clinical Investigation* 4 (1997): 1129–1133.

3. J.R. Hibbeln, "Fish Consumption and Major Depression." *The Lancet* 351 (1998): 1213.

4. J.R. Hibbeln et al., "Dietary Polyunsaturated Fatty Acids and Depression: When Cholesterol Does Not Satisfy," *American Journal of Clinical Nutrition* 62 (1995): 1–9.

5. J. Carper, *Your Miracle Brain* (New York: HarperCollins, 2000): 78.

6. N.L. Mace and P.V. Rabins, *The 36-Hour Day* (New York: Warner, 2001): 184–189.

7. Ibid., 35.

8. J.C. Rogers et al., "Improving Morning Care Routines of Nursing Home Residents with Dementia," *Journal of the American Geriatrics Society* 47, no. 9: 1049–1057.

9. J. Medina, *What You Need to Know About Alzheimer's Disease* (Hong Kong: CME and New Harbinger, 1999): 130.

10. F. Gray-Davidson, *Alzheimer's Disease: Frequently Asked Questions: Making Sense of the Journey* (Los Angeles: Lowell House, 1999): 151.

11. L.S. Berk et al., "Neuroendocrine and Stress Hormone Changes During Mirthful Laughter," *American Journal of Medical Science* 298 (1989): 390–396.

12. C. Peterson et al., "Pessimistic Explanatory Style Is a Risk Factor for Illness: A 35-Year Longitudinal Study," *Journal of Personality and Social Psychology* 55 (1988): 23–27.

13. N. Cousins, "Anatomy of an Illness (As Perceived by the Patient)," *New England Journal of Medicine* 295 (1979): 1458–1463.

14. C.J. Charnetski and F.X. Brennan, *Feeling Good Is Good for You: How Pleasure Can Boost Your Immune System and Lengthen Your Life* (Emmaus, PA: Rodale, 2001): 51.

15. Ibid., 55.

16. Ibid., 56.

Chapter 6

1. N.L. Mace and P.V. Rabins, *The 36-Hour Day* (New York: Warner, 2001): 381.

2. S.M. Bell, *Visiting Mom, an Unexpected Gift* (Sedona, AZ: Elder, 2000).

3. *USA Today*, May 17, 1993: 1D–2D.

4. "Steps to Understanding Financial Issues: Resources for Individuals with Alzheimer's Disease," Alzheimer's Association Action Series (Chicago: Alzheimer's Association).

Chapter 7

1. D. Snowdon, *Aging with Grace* (New York: Bantam, 2001): 14.

2. Ibid., 185.

3. Ibid., 113.

4. Ibid., 38.

5. Ibid., 95.

6. Ibid., 193–194.

7. Alzheimer's Association, "Education May Protect Against Alzheimer's Disease and Other Forms of Dementia," reporting on a study presented at the World Alzheimer's Disease Congress 2000 by Margaret Gatz, Ph.D., professor of psychology at the University of Southern California, Los Angeles, www.alz.org/media/news/current/educationmayprotect.htm, accessed December, 16, 2001.

8. R.P. Friedland et al., *Proceedings of the National Academy of Sciences*, www.theage.com.au/entartainment/2001/03/07/FFX7FXPGYJC.html, accessed December 8, 2001.

9. Ibid.

10. Ibid.

11. H. Van Praag et al., "Running Enhances Neurogenesis, Learning and Long-Term Potentiation in Mice," *Proceedings of the National Academy of Sciences (USA)* 96, no. 23 (1999): 13427–13431.

12. National Institute on Aging and National Institutes of Health, *2000 Progress Report on Alzheimer's Disease*, NIH Publication no. 00-4859 (Washington, D.C.: Government Printing Office, 2000): 28.

13. Friedland et al., *Proceedings of the National Academy of Sciences*.

14. Snowdon, *Aging with Grace*: 38.

15. D.H. Smith, *Journal of Neuropathology and Experimental Neurology* (September 1999), www.lahaaland.com/science/medicine/medicine126.html, accessed December 9, 2001.

16. Ibid.

17. Snowdon, *Aging with Grace*: 181.

18. J. Carper, *Your Miracle Brain* (New York: HarperCollins, 2000): 152–153.

19. M. Sano et al., "A Controlled Trial of Selegeline, Alpha-Tocopherol or Both as Treatments for Alzheimer's Disease," *New England Journal of Medicine* 336 (1997): 1216–1222.

20. Mark A. Sager, "Preventing Alzheimer's Disease," Wisconsin Department of Health and Family Services, www.dhfs.state.wi.us/aging/age_news/NO114/ALZprev.htm, accessed December 4, 2001.

21. Ibid.

22. Snowdon, *Aging with Grace*: 179.

23. R. Clarke et al., "Folate, Vitamin B_{12} and Serum Homocysteine Levels in Confirmed Alzheimer's Disease," *Archives of Neurology* 55 (1998): 1449–1455.

24. Carper, *Your Miracle Brain*: 311.

25. S. Seshadri et al., "Plasma Homocysteine As a Risk Factor for Dementia and Alzheimer's Disease," *New England Journal of Medicine*, February 14, 2002, 346(7): 466–468.

26. "High Homocysteine Levels May Double Risk of Dementia, Alzheimer's Disease, New Report Suggests," The National Institutes of Health press release, www.nih.gov/news/pr/feb2002/nia-13.htm, accessed March 16, 2002.

27. S. Frautschy, from a study presented at the annual meeting of the Society of Neuroscience in San Diego, CA, November 15, 2001, as reported

by Reuters's Health Information, www.nlm.nih.gov/medlineplus?news?
fullstory_4754.html, accessed December 14, 2001.

28. Ibid.

29. Ibid.

30. R.L. Prior, "Antioxidant Capacity and Polyphenolic Components of Teas: Implications for Altering In Vivo Antioxidant Status," *Proceedings of the Society for Experimental Biology and Medicine* 220, no. 4 (1999): 255–261.

31. "Wine," Alzheimer's Association, www.alz.org/media/positions/wine.htm, accessed November 20, 2001.

32. Snowdon, *Aging with Grace:* 173.

33. Carper, *Your Miracle Brain:* 163.

34. D. Kuhn, *Alzheimer's Early Stages* (Alameda, CA: Hunter House, 1999): 52.

35. Carper, *Your Miracle Brain:* 73.

36. Snowdon, *Aging with Grace:* 164.

37. W.A. Kukall et al., "Solvent Exposure As a Risk Factor for Alzheimer's Disease: A Case-Control Study," *American Journal of Epidemiology* 141, no. 11 (1995): 1059–1071.

38. Kuhn, *Alzheimer's Early Stages:* 53.

39. E. Sobel et al., "Elevated Risk of Alzheimer's Disease Among Workers with Likely Electromagnetic Field Exposure," *Neurology* 47, no. 6 (1996): 1477–1481.

40. C.E. Greenwood et al., "Cognitive Impairment in Rats Fed High-Fat Diets: A Specific Effect of Saturated Fatty Acid Intake," *Behavioral Neuroscience* 110 (1996): 451–459.

41. Carper, *Your Miracle Brain:* 61.

42. Ibid., 333–334.

43. E.L. Helkala et al., "Midlife Vascular Risk Factors and Alzheimer's Disease in Later Life: Longitudinal Population-Based Study," *British Medical Journal* 322 (2001): 1447–1451.

44. S. Seiner, "High Blood Pressure and High Cholesterol in Midlife May Increase Risks of Alzheimer's Disease," Vertitas Medicine for Patients, Alzheimer's Disease, Viewpoint Archives, www.veritasmedicine.com/archives.cfm?did=1&mode=2&item_id=1532, accessed November 19, 2001.

45. "Cholesterol: A Clue to Alzheimer's?" HealthAtoZ.com, www.healthatoz.com/atoz/HealthUpdate/alert11022000.html, accessed December 9, 2001.

46. B. Wolozin et al., "Decreased Prevalence of Alzheimer's Disease Associated with 3-Hydroxy-3-methyglutaryl Coenzyme A Reductase Inhibitors," *Archives of Neurology* 57 (2000): 1459.

47. L.M. Refolo et al., "Hypercholesterolemia Accelerates the Alzheimer's Amyloid Pathology in Transgenic Mouse Model," *Neurobiology of Disease* 7, no. 21 (2000).

Chapter 8

1. K. Garb, "An End to Alzheimer's?" *Technology Review* (March 2001): 77.

2. D. Shenk, *The Forgetting—Alzheimer's: Portrait of an Epidemic* (New York: Doubleday, 2001): 158.

3. Ibid., 159.

4. Ibid., 187–188.

5. Garb, "An End to Alzheimer's?": 73

6. National Institute on Aging and National Institutes of Health, *2000 Progress Report on Alzheimer's Disease*, NIH Publication no. 00-4859 (Washington, D.C.: Government Printing Office, 2000): 9.

7. Garb, "An End to Alzheimer's?": 73.

8. D. Christensen, "Attacking Alzheimer's: Comprehending the Causes Gets More Complex," *Science News* 160 (2001): 286.

9. Ibid.

10. Ibid.

11. Ibid.

12. Ibid.

13. J. Lewis et al., "Enhanced Neurofibrillary Degeneration in Transgenic Mice Expressing Mutant Tau and APP," *Science* 293, August 24, 2001: 1487–1491.

14. Christensen, "Attacking Alzheimer's": 287.

15. Garb, "An End to Alzheimer's?": 72.

16. Ibid., 74.

17. Ibid.

18. Ibid., 73.

19. Ibid., 75.

20. "Experimental Therapy May Be Useful in Treating and Preventing Alzheimer's Disease," Elan Corporation press release July 23, 2001, www.elancorp.com, accessed November 16, 2001.

21. C. Janus et al., "Ae Peptide Immunization Reduces Behavioral Impairment and Plaques in a Model of Alzheimer's Disease," *Nature* 408 (2000).

22. "Alzheimer's Disease Immunotherapeutic to Advance to Exploratory Phase 2A Studies," Elan Corporation press release July 23, 2001, News Room, www.elancorp.com, accessed November 16, 2001.

23. R. Rowland, "Alzheimer's Vaccine Passes Key Test," July 23, 2001, CNN.com, www.cnn.com, accessed December 7, 2001.

24. "NeoTherapeutics' Neotrofin Stimulates Proliferation of Neural Stem Cells in Adult Mice," NeoTherapeutics press release, November 16, 2001, www.neot.com, accessed December 11, 2001.

25. J. Fischer, "The First Clone," *US News & World Report* (December 3, 2001): 58–60.

26. Christensen, "Attacking Alzheimer's": 287.

27. C. Ezzell, "The Stem Cell Show Stopper?" *Scientific American* 285, no. 6 (2001): 27.

28. Tanzi and Parson, *Decoding Darkness:* 191–195.

29. W. Daw et al., "The Number of Trait Loci in Late-Onset Alzheimer Disease," *American Journal of Human Genetics* 66, no. 1 (2000): 196–204.

30. Tanzi and Parson, *Decoding Darkness:* 220.

31. "Abstract Titles of Research Funded in 2001," Alzheimer's Association, www.alz.org, accessed December 11, 2001.

32. B. De Strooper and G. Koning, "Alzheimer's Disease: An Inflammatory Drug Prospect," *Nature* 414 (2001): 159–160.

33. R.K. Sobel, "Memory Pill," *US News & World Report* (November 19, 2001): 59.

34. D. DeNoon, "Metal Remover Clears Alzheimer's Plaques in Mice—But Will It Improve Disease Symptoms?" WebMD Medical News, November 28, 2001, www.webmd.com, accessed December 2, 2001.

35. Ibid.

36. R. Rowland, "Cholesterol Drug May Prevent Alzheimer's," CNN.com, www.cnn.com, accessed December 5, 2001.

37. Ibid.

38. *2000 Progress Report on Alzheimer's Disease:* 11–12.

39. D.P. Perl et al., "Alzheimer's Disease and Parkinson's Disease: Distinct Entities or Extremes of a Spectrum of Neurodegeneration?" *Annuals of Neurology* 44, no. 3 (1998).

40. *2000 Progress Report on Alzheimer's Disease:* 23.

41. Ibid.

42. Ibid., 12.

43. Ibid., 12–13.
44. "Human Genome Project," U.S. Department of Energy, www.ornl.gov /hgmis, accessed December 14, 2001.
45. Tanzi and Parson, *Decoding Darkness:* 202–203.

Glossary

acetylcholine   A brain chemical (neurotransmitter) important for the transmission of nerve signals responsible for learning and memory, which is in short supply in people with Alzheimer's disease.

activities of daily living (ADLs)   Basic activities such as dressing, eating, bathing, and using the toilet that can become difficult for people in the later stages of Alzheimer's disease to perform.

adult day care   Facilities providing therapeutic services as well as recreational activities for older adults with a variety of disabilities, not just dementia.

agnosia   An early but unusual symptom of Alzheimer's disease characterized by difficulty judging spatial distances or recognizing familiar objects or people.

amyloid   *See* beta-amyloid.

amyloid plaques   Deposits consisting of beta-amyloid protein plus dead and dying brain cells thought to be at least partially responsible for AD's symptoms.

amyloid precursor protein (APP)   A naturally occurring protein in the body from which beta-amyloid—a major component of AD's amyloid plaques—is thought to be formed.

anti-inflammatories   Medications such as ibuprofen, naproxen sodium, aspirin, and prescription drugs known as COX-2 inhibitors that some research indicates may help reduce AD risks.

antioxidants   Substances in the body that help protect cells from being damaged by naturally occurring by-products of metabolism called free radicals.

ApoE4   Gene thought to increase risks of developing Alzheimer's disease.

assisted living facility   Apartment-style living quarters in which assistance with daily tasks is provided, including meals, but not medical care.

autopsy   An examination of the human body or one of its organs done after death.

axon   A tentacle-like portion of a neuron (brain cell) responsible for the transmission (as opposed to reception) of nerve impulses.

behavioral symptoms   Behaviors caused by Alzheimer's disease such as agitation, wandering, repeated questions, and physical aggression that can be troublesome for caregivers to manage.

beta-amyloid   A protein that collects to form dense deposits in the brain, called amyloid plaques, that are thought to cause Alzheimer's disease by leading to the destruction of brain cells in their vicinity.

blood brain barrier   A vascular network that serves to protect the brain from potentially harmful foreign substances.

capillaries   The smallest branches of the body's blood vessel system responsible for nourishing cells on an individual level.

caregiver   A person responsible for the physical and emotional well-being of someone who is physically or mentally impaired.

cell   The smallest unit of a living organism capable of functioning on its own.

cerebral cortex   The area of the brain most involved in higher thought processes such as learning, language, and reasoning.

cholinesterase inhibitors   Medications that help maintain cognitive function by helping preserve levels of a neurotransmitter called acetylcholine.

chromosomes   Threadlike structures within the nucleus of a cell that exist in 23 pairs (one from mom, one from dad) and that contain the material (DNA) that comprise the genes.

clinical trial   A carefully controlled study designed to test whether a treatment or drug is safe and effective for human use.

cognitive function   The ability to perform a higher mental process such as speaking, reading, reasoning, remembering, and making judgments.

computerized tomography scan (CT or CAT scan)   A diagnostic test that uses a computer along with x-rays to produce a highly detailed picture of the physical structure of the brain.

dementia   A term broadly used to refer to any condition whereby normal mental capabilities suffer from a decline due to organic causes.

dendrites   Tentacle-like projections of neurons that serve to receive (rather than transmit) nerve signals from other brain cells.

DNA (deoxyribonucleic acid)   Molecules within the body's chromosomes that, in paired sequences, comprise the genes.

estrogen   A naturally occurring hormone that some studies indicate may reduce risks of Alzheimer's disease in women when given to them following menopause.

familial Alzheimer's disease (FAD)   A rare type of Alzheimer's disease that appears to be inherited and that occurs in two forms—early-onset (striking people as young as 30 to 40) and late-onset (occurring in people 60 and older). FAD has been estimated to constitute about 5 percent of all AD cases, most (about 95 percent) being of the late-onset variety.

folic acid (also called folate)   A nutrient prevalent in leafy green vegetables that some studies suggest may help prevent AD's onset.

free radicals   Highly toxic molecules that are produced naturally in the body by a process known as oxidation; thought to be a risk for causing AD and many other diseases as well as the aging process itself.

geriatrician   A medical doctor specializing in treating the elderly.

Ginkgo biloba   An extract from the leaves of the ginkgo tree that some research suggests may help treat AD as well as reduce risks of its onset.

hippocampus   An area of the brain responsible for memory and one of the first that Alzheimer's disease affects.

huperzine-A   A dietary supplement derived from a type of Chinese moss that has chemical properties and medicinal effects similar to cholinesterase inhibitors in helping improve cognitive function.

inflammation   A reaction by the body to injury or infection that some research suggests may play a role in how Alzheimer's disease develops.

magnetic resonance imaging (MRI)   A diagnostic technique that uses magnetic fields to produce computer images of the brain's anatomy as well as activity.

metabolism   The process whereby the body converts food into energy.

nerve growth factor (NGF)   Molecules that some scientists theorize may help protect brain cells from being destroyed by AD's amyloid plaques.

neurofibrillary tangles   Abnormal structures found inside some of the brain cells of people with Alzheimer's disease that can kill the cells by causing a collapse of their skeletal structure.

neuron   A nerve cell in the brain and a target of AD's destructive forces.

neuroscientist   A scientist specializing in the study of the brain.

neurotransmitter   A chemical messenger that is released by the axon of one nerve cell in the brain and picked up by the dendrite of another, thus forming the chemical foundation of human thought.

power of attorney   A legal arrangement whereby responsibility for decisions affecting a person's financial or physical well-being is granted to another person.

positron emission tomography (PET)   An imaging procedure that measures brain activity by monitoring the brain's blood flow as well as its use of oxygen and glucose.

protease   An enzyme that splits proteins into smaller particles.

receptor   A protein within a cell that recognizes and binds to chemical messengers such as neurotransmitters.

respite care   Temporary relief from the burdens of caregiving provided either in the home or at an outside facility.

serotonin   A neurotransmitter lacking in people with AD, low levels of which also are associated with depression.

single photon emission computerized tomography (SPECT)   An imaging technique that measures blood flow to different parts of the brain.

special care unit   A long-term care facility specifically designed for the needs of people with dementia.

sundowning   The tendency for behavioral symptoms of Alzheimer's disease to get worse in the late afternoon and early evening.

synapse   The minute space between nerve cells across which nerve impulses carried by neurotransmitters must pass.

tau   A protein within neurons that in people with AD begins to form stick-like structures (filaments) that become the neurofibrillary tangles causing nerve cells to die.

vitamin E   An antioxidant that some research suggests may help prevent Alzheimer's disease and/or slow its progression by reducing damage to brain cells caused by toxic molecules called free radicals.

Index

A

Acetylcholine
  cholinesterase inhibitors and, 68–73
  defined, 7, 67–68
  estrogen and, 87
Acquired Immune Deficiency
    Syndrome (AIDS), 62
Adult day care centers, 190–191
African Americans, 27
Age as risk factor, 21
Aging versus AD, 19
Agitation, treating, 84
Alcohol
  as hazard, 126, 146
  red wine, 222–224
Aluminum, 24, 226–227
Alzheimer, Dr. Alois, 1, 3–6
Alzheimer's Association
  as caregiver's best friend, 177
  clinical trial information from, 75
  HELPLINE, 46
  legal concerns and, 199
  local branches, 56
  support groups and, 175
Alzheimer's disease (AD). *See also*
    Diagnosis; Prevention of AD
  aging versus, 19
  causes of, 19–21, 213–214
  conditions that mimic, 60–62
  death and, 12, 18–19

discovery of, 3–7
mild cognitive impairment (MCI)
    versus, 51, 254
as progressive disease, 103
risk factors for, 21–27
sporadic versus familial, 26
stages of, 57–60
statistics on, 12–13
symptoms of, 7–18
treatments for, 65–100
in women, 12, 23, 86–88
Amygdala, defined, 144
Amyloid hypothesis. *See* Beta-amyloid
    theory
Amyloid plaque. *See also* Treatments for
    suspected causes
  defined, 5, 9, 237
  tau tangles and, 238–239
Angiogenesis
  defined, 222
  green tea and, 221–222, 250
  research on, 246–251
Angry caregivers. *See also* Caregivers
  guilt in, 164, 177–178
  as hazard, 126
  stress and, 164, 167
Antidepressants, 26, 82–83
Anti-inflammatory medications
  angiogenesis and, 250
  as treatment, 85–86, 251, 257

About the Author

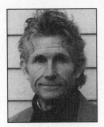

Porter Shimer has been a health and fitness journalist since graduating from Princeton University with a B.A. in English literature in 1971. In addition to 11 books, including *New Hope for People with Diabetes*, he has written a nationally syndicated newspaper column, newsletters, and articles for *Prevention, Ladies Home Journal, Mode, Reader's Digest* and *Men's Health*. The father of two daughters—Elizabeth, 26, and Sarah, 20—he lives in Emmaus, Pennsylvania with his wife, Claire, and 2-year-old son and office mate, Michael.

About the Reviewers

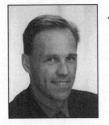

Juergen H. A. Bludau, M.D., C.M.D., is a board-certified fellowship-trained geriatrician and the medical director for the Joseph L. Morse Geriatric Center and its affiliate agencies, the Institute for Geriatric Research & Training and the Lola & Saul Kramer Senior Services Agency in West Palm Beach, Florida. Dr. Bludau is a voluntary assistant professor of medicine at the University of Miami Medical School, an Instructor on Medicine at Harvard Medical School and, in 2001, was appointed to the Alzheimer's Disease Advisory Committee by Governor Jeb Bush. Dr. Bludau lives in West Palm Beach, Florida, with his wife, Paola, and their three children.

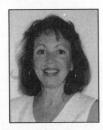

Avrene L. Brandt, Ph.D., is a clinical psychologist with a private practice in Wallingford, Pennsylvania, and a consultant to the Greater Philadelphia Chapter of the Alzheimer's Association and to geriatric and rehabilitation facilities in Pennsylvania, Delaware, and New Jersey. Dr. Brandt is the author of *Caregiver's Reprieve*. She lives in Wallingford, Pennsylvania.

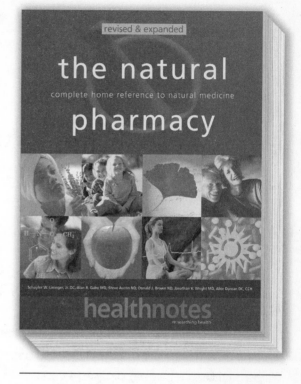

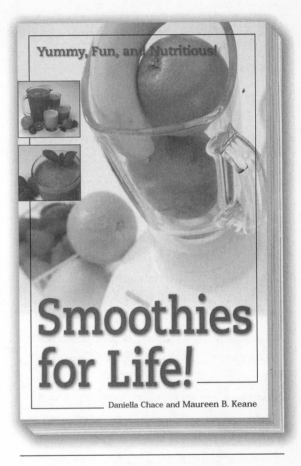